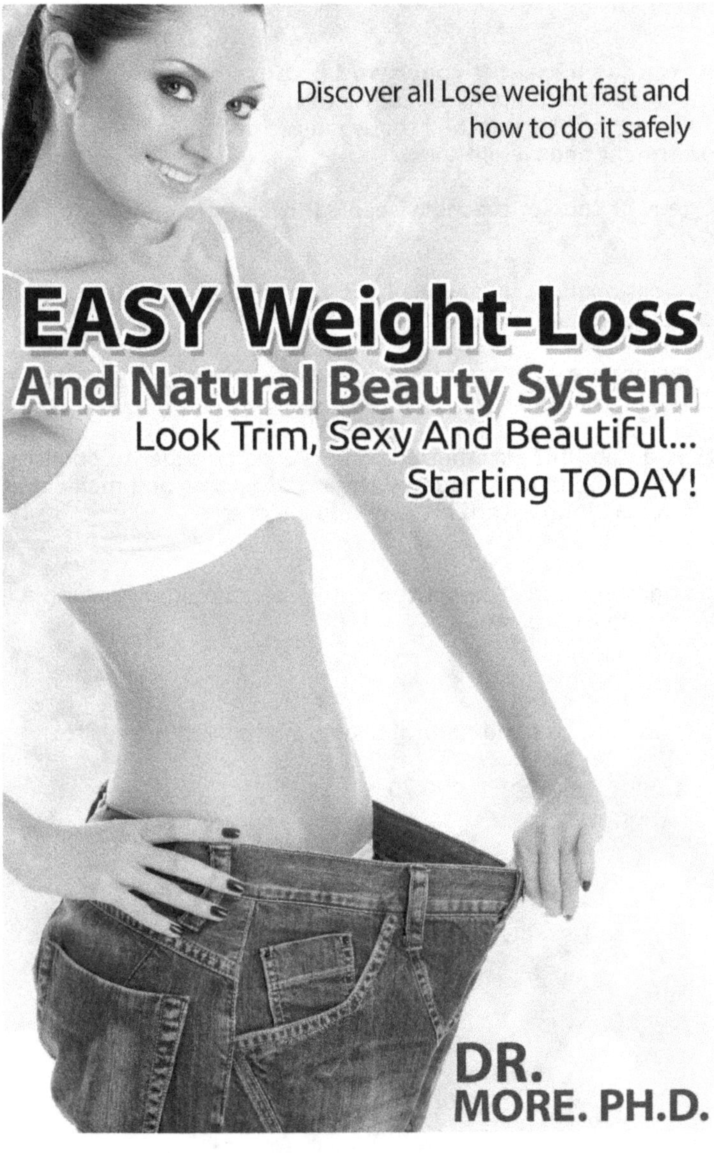

Discover all Lose weight fast and
how to do it safely

EASY Weight-Loss
And Natural Beauty System
Look Trim, Sexy And Beautiful...
Starting TODAY!

DR.
MORE. PH.D.

About The Author

Dr. Morgan is a master coach and professional trainer. He has trained corporate companies like, Microsoft, IBM, etc in corporate team building. He has also coached thousands of people in personal empowerment and weight-loss.

His forte is of course, coaching people in weight-loss and natural beauty!

As a professional coach/trainer, he is accredited by the International Accreditation Institute-USA.

His ancestors are from India and Fiji Islands, they finally settled in beautiful Malaysia.

He is the author of four other books. He is no stranger to publicity, having appeared in numerous TV shows, programs and media. He now lives in Kuala Lumpur with his wife and children.

He manages and runs a weight-loss membership program with a like minded group of experts

Author's weight-loss and natural beauty membership website:

www.weightloss-expert-group.com

"The Last Weight-loss Plan You Will Ever Need"

The Mediterranean Diet, The Atkins Diet, South Beach Diet, Zone Diet, Cabbage Soup Diet, Negative Calorie Diet! Geesh, it's enough to drive you straight to the grocery store for a pint of Ben and Jerry's finest!

Have you tried some or all of those diets? Are you sick and tired of being pushed, shoved and pulled in 10 different directions when it comes to finding a diet that works?

Your Search Is Over!

Ready, get set, GO! Let's work together And ***Burn Calories"*** today and lose your first few pounds tomorrow!

Let's Go!

TABLE OF CONTENTS

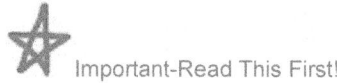

The Last Weight-loss Program You Will Ever Need

INTRODUCTION

If you struggle with weight gain it's a good bet that you have tried at least one of the "fad" diets that crop up on a regular basis.

The truth is that some of these diets may grant you temporary weight loss. In the usual case, however, the weight returns as soon as you stray from the diet.

The bottom line is that you gain weight because you consume more calories than your body is able to use and no diet is a substitute for good eating habits.

Your body requires a certain amount of calories in order to function properly. If you truly wish to lose weight you must burn off more calories than your body requires.

In this guide you will learn ways to reduce the amount of calories you ingest as well as tips and techniques to help you burn off unnecessary calories.

Before we begin, however, it's important that you fill your arsenal with every possible tool available to insure your success. The most important tool in your weight loss program does not include diet or exercise.

There is no special equipment you need to purchase. You don't need to join a gym or health club. And, you already have every component you need to put this tool to work for you and begin a successful weight loss program. What

We have also included some very workable secret processes that will accelerate your weight-loss! Having said that, let's get started, shall we?

* VERY IMPORTANT! *

Read this very carefully.

As you read look out for this symbol…the star! It's very important. It stands for VERY IMPORTANT PRACTICAL TIPS YOU CAN USE FOR FAST RESULTS! If you want to browse and look for the star and just read the SPECIAL practical tips, it;s okay, after that come back and read through the whole book to get the complete picture…Okay!

Now enjoy your reading…see you slim!

In our sales page we promised you instant tips for easy weight-loss. Well, before we start off with the main program…here it is!

FAST TRACK TIPS.

TIP NO.1. You can lose an average of 15 to 25 lbs per year without doing anything! All you need to do is cut off soft drinks from your normal diet, that's all! If you, say consumer about 3 cans of soft drinks a day, and you stop doing that you WILL lose all those lbs. Replace your normal diet of sodas with mineral water or fresh fruit juices!

TIP NO.2. Re-learn to breathe! In the chapters below we will be giving

some very special breathing exercises under YOGA BREATHING, chose 2 you

find comfortable. Do one in the morning before breakfast and one in the evening

before dinner. These breathing methods will help burn off TOXINS (one of the

main causes of excess fat) and reduce weight. These breathing methods must

be done comfortably, do not strain!

Low energy and weight gain is not a natural part of our life, these are symptoms of a metabolic imbalance, what medical doctors call 'insulin resistance syndrome', which can, if not addressed, lead to diabetes and heart disease.

Anytime you eat carbohydrate foods, like bread, potatoes, chips, pastries, pasta, rice and sweets, it is converted into sugar by your body during digestion. In order to now use this sugar up as fuel, your body releases a hormone called insulin needed by your cells to convert the sugar into energy.

Because the modern diet is mostly made up of carbohydrates and/or refined sugar, your body's cells start to become _insensitive_ to your own insulin. In other words, your cells start to **resist** your body's own insulin.

Without this natural balance the insulin being resisted _signals_ your body to _store sugar as fat_, this shifts your metabolism into the fat saving mode. Your metabolism slows down and makes it _impossible_ for you to lose weight no matter how hard you try. That's why you're always **tired** and **hungry**

That's the reason why lots of people, keep gaining back weight from fat.

Now there is now something you can do about it, once and for all. The answer is to attack the root cause of weight gain by providing your body what it needs to replenish itself at the cellular level, thereby balancing your body's metabolism. This solution is absolutely safe and natural...DEEP YOGA BREATHING. (See book on Yoga below).

TIP NO.3. Burn calories while eating normally! Yes you can! Break

down your 3 times a day meals into 5 times a day routine. Break your meals into smaller portions and eat 5 meals. Eg…Breakfast, Morning Tea, Lunch, Evening Tea and Dinner before 7.00 to 7.30 pm and don't eat anything after that. If you do feel hungry, just take a couple of thin slices of whole meal bread…And drink a lot of water in before meals.

TIP NO.4. Scientists have discovered that stress is the likely cause of stubborn belly fat.

According to government researchers, the link between stress, tension, and **excess belly fat** is clear. High levels of **cortisol stress hormone** can cause pound after pound of excess body fat to accumulate around your waist and tummy, a condition affecting millions of people… mostly women.

(We have added a special section on STRESS too. The moment you have learned to relax while doing normal everyday chores and work related activities half your battle of the BULGE is won!).

But most important…here is a dynamic secret method that will instantly bring down your stress level and your weight.

HERE IT IS… Every person has a center of gravity in his body, as does all objects. Your center is located about two inches below the navel. For simplicity's sake we will call it the 'center' in this discussion, okay? All humans have this center located just below the navel (About 2 inches below). . To enable total relaxation, and DE-STRES, you must put your concentration in this spot, and relax yourself.

Let me also show you a simple breathing exercise that you can utilize while you concentrate on your center, which will help burn calories at the same time.

For this breathing procedure you must breathe in through the nose and out through the mouth. As you breathe in, imagine your breath going in straight to a point ten inches behind your head. As you do this you will find that your head automatically tilts back. As your head tilts back, simultaneously feel your center (two inches below your navel) expanding.

Hold it for a count of six and breathe out. You can do it as many times as you like. Its safe, it's simple and that's all there is to it. One important thing you must never forget is, your breathing must be gradual, slow, smooth and comfortable. By dropping your concentration to the center and combining it with your breathing you can achieve oneness of body and mind. You can harness the benefits of body / mind integration which will enable you to have total relaxation with regular practice.

==== YOUR BOOK STARTS NOW! ====

ATTITUDE.

 After reading through ATTITUDE, follow the scrip below to enhance and accelerate your weight-loss!

SCRIPT FOR WEIGHT_LOSS!

(This is an ancient metaphysical principle. I have made it easy and workable by modifying it to modern times. It is a powerful system. I call it, 'Auranetics®'.

AURANETICS® PERSONAL EMPOWERMENT PROGRAM.
Auranetics® is the science of creating and internalizing an aura of personal power using your subconscious mind. You put in place personal power modules and get rid of your negative traits.

Here in this particular instance we are discussing weight-loss. Below is how *Auranetics®* is used to manage weight and other positive values. You can modify and use *Auranetics®* throughout the book to address particular issues at hand.

AURANETICS® PERSONAL EMPOWERMENT PROGRAM- SUBJECT:

The Last Weight-loss Program You Will Ever Need

Losing weight and looking good.

How is your internal dialog today?
(Here tell yourself frankly how being overweight affects you. Here is an example I have used)

"Negative. I feel nervous. From the time I got up, I feel a lump in my throat. I can recognize it…feeling of negativity. I feel I am overweight. I don't look slim and sexy. I feel no one will take notice of me, maybe except to notice the way I dress, like a slob, as usual! "

My new empowered script…
(Fill in your new empowered outlook on YOUR PROBLEM and relate it to your particular action or life episode. You can modify it to suit any and all instruction in this book. God Bless! Here is to a new SLIM, DYNAMIC YOU!).

"There is nothing to feel negative about this issue of being overweight. It happens to a lot of people. Most don't do anything about it…BUT. I am taking responsibility and DOING something about IT…Something POSSITIVE! "

THIS IS A 'DYNAMIC IMAGE PROJECTION'® DESTINY SERIES.

Your personal Movie-"I am the master of my destiny"…Part one-'The NEW YOU'.

You are the hero/heroine in this movie. Let me give you an outline. You produce the movie. You direct it. Add music, special effects and dialog. Do it after I have given you the outline of the story. You are free to modify any area of the movie to fit your personal needs. After all, you are the director of your life and producer of your personal destiny…AND THE HEROINE!

The outline.

'The alarm rings. You get up excited about the day ahead. You roll over, kiss you husband/ wife. "Good morning darling." You murmur into his/ her ears.

The Last Weight-loss Program You Will Ever Need

You jump up from bed, walk to the bathroom. You wash up and look into the mirror. You smile. The image smiles back at you. It looks confident and strong. You feel great!

You believe in yourself…you want to look good in:

- *in your jeans*
- *not get out of breath*
- *feel more confident*
- *enjoy shopping new attire, that will compliment your new slim look*
- *have more ZEST and energy for living*
- *feel good about yourself, the new YOU!*

You walk back into the bedroom, pull on your track bottoms, your 'T' shirt, and walk down to the front. You put on your running shoes, do a few stretches.

While stretching, you keep your mind on track. You tell yourself, 'I feel good. I am a loving powerful and passionate lady. I am feeling fine and in perfect health, feeling better than before.' You stretched yourself and did a few TRIGGERS, while you stretched.

You go back to your room, feeling great and exhilarated. Feeling confident and in charge. You get ready to go to work.

While driving your kids to school, you are calm. You are listening to a light inspirational music. As you near your office, you think about how you are going to face your day, as a new person. You stomach knots in fear for a few seconds. The adrenalin rushes through your system.

Amid your fear, you turn the negative feelings around. You experience the thrill, exhilaration and excitement of the new dynamic personality you are creating for yourself. It's a challenge for you…But you know you will win. You are confident you will be able to lose the appropriate weight, improve your outlook. You tell yourself, this new personality you are creating for yourself will bring tremendous value to not only you personally but to your family as well.

Your confidence, in your new personal project shows through, your smile is radiant and is noticed by all!

End of outline.

You are in charge NOW! Take over.

Now that you have the outline, can you go and sit in the director's chair please, and direct this movie? Give it your best. You are now the famous director-Spielberg! (Or whoever is your favorite.)

Use your imagination, your visualization. Picture the scenario, capture the impressions, the emotions, and characterize it. Add special effects and inspirational music, where appropriate. Remember you are the heroine, so build in a self-image of a dynamic slim, beautiful personality.

WANT ME TO GIVE YOU AN EXAMPLE? HERE IT IS BELOW!

Sample personal movie…In this movie your name is SALLY!

"You are dressed to go out! You have selected the best you have, the new model jeans you have not worn for sometimes, that you bought just after your wedding, when you were slimmer… You walk holding you body and neck straight, relaxed, like a model on a catwalk.

(Add your favorite music here!)

As you walk into the office, everyone turns around. You smile a greeting. You look different today…You are looking radiant, you have lost some weight and you look great in that jeans. You look beautiful!

(Add more music here!)

"Sally, you are looking GREAT!" your friends exclaim. You smile and say thank you. Everybody is noticing you, the new you!

After work you reach home…your husband walks out and hugs you. "You look GREEEAT DARLING" he whispers.

^^^^^^^^

Okay, that's it. Now use your imagination, your visualization and picture all these in your mind.

Do know why this works and has brought weight-loss and other benefits to many? Simply because, your subconscious mind works on this subtle suggestions and channels, BELIEVES IT A 100 % and then simultaneously directs your conscious mind, which in turn, directs you, your body to act so.

Have you heard about, "'ACT AS IF' and IT WILL BECOME"? It's true, and has worked for hundreds of years!

Have you heard about the, 'Act Thin, Be Thin' movement? It is a hit, it's based on these premise.

So, my dear friend, believe and it will be so. They say believe can move mountains, but in our case, it can help to shed a few pounds and sculpt a new you!

A famous Russian, psychiatrist Dr. Vladimir Raikov, developed a breakthrough to enhance personal development called, 'Artificial Reincarnation' an exciting methodology where participants take the role of people with special talents. In this program, participants select model subjects they want to 'role play'. In NLP a similar module called 'MODELLING' is used.

Say for example, Jane Fonda is a subject for a wholesome, beautiful, slim woman. You want to take her as a subject…then you need to go into, 'Artificial Reincarnation', and model after Jane Fonda, meaning, 'REINCARNATE ARTIFICIALY' into being Jane Fonda, meaning, be HER. How does she stand, how does she speak, what she does successfully, what type of exercises, etc.

==========okay, lets continue=============

Once you have done that, relax, close your eyes. Sit in a quiet place where you will not be disturbed and play back this completed movie.

Internalize it. This is how you will operate from now on. Negativity will not affect you anymore.

You will modify this script, make a new movie, to suit another 'Weight-loss, Natural Beauty' situation and take the role of the HERO/HEROINE!

Continue With ATTITUDE…

If you have tried every diet on the planet, every exercise program from the latest fitness guru and repeatedly failed to achieve your weight loss goals you probably need a "check up from the neck up."

Successful weight loss doesn't just happen. It took more than a few months to reach the point where you are at right now. Give yourself a break and expect it to take awhile before you see measurable results. Take a leap of faith and follow some basic principles.

Begin with your "self talk." This is the conversation that runs through your brain continuously. What kind of conversation do you have with your self talk? What type of negative self talk has kept you from reaching your goals in the past?

If you had a chance to do it over again, would you change the dialogue? That's a no-brainer isn't it? Well, the good news is that you can turn the tide of negative self talk beginning right now. It's never too late to begin and you start by reprogramming your self talk.

A good starting point is to begin with positive affirmations. Positive affirmations spoken aloud with authority and belief, positively affect your attitude, focuses your thinking and lead to a course of action that will help you become the person you want to be and have the things that you want to have.

Begin by writing your affirmations on paper. You need to take some time for this exercise. You can begin with something like, "I want to lose 25 pounds before Christmas." That's a worthy goal and attainable, but we need to put some work into structuring the affirmation.

First of all, "I want" gives the impression that what you desire is always in the future. In order to re-program your self-talk, you need to trick your mind into believing that you have already achieved success. This is how your subconscious mind functions.

Your subconscious mind has no capacity for understanding the concept of time. Everything is in the moment . . . here and now. When you tell your subconscious mind that you "want" that is exactly what you will get . . .want. . .without ever achieving fulfillment. Unless you change your mental tape recorder, you will achieve exactly what you are telling your subconscious, that you "want to lose 25 pounds." You will "want to lose 25 pounds" for the rest of your days unless you change your self talk.

If your weight is 150 pounds and you desire is to weight 125 pounds, then you need to "be" 125 pounds from the moment you make the decision to change your self talk.

What if you write your affirmation to read something like this: **"I am healthy and fit weighing 125 pounds."**

What are you telling your subconscious now? It's extremely important that you phrase your affirmation as if you have already accomplished what you desire. Work on writing it out until you have it precisely as you wish to become.

It is extremely important that your affirmation is crystal clear because what you affirm is exactly what your subconscious mind will bring you.

You needn't limit yourself to one affirmation either. Write another one that reflects your new exercise program. "I enjoy my healthy new exercise program," or, "I love the healthy foods I eat."

Write and rewrite until you are absolutely certain that you have written your goals "in the here and now" AND represent precisely what you desire. Only then do you begin to speak it aloud and do so several times a day.

Remember to use the present tense. "I acknowledge achievement in all my weight loss goals." "I have the skill and talent to exercise every day." "I am a winner." "I am grateful for all of my accomplishments no matter how small."

At first you will feel awkward and uncomfortable and you may not feel or believe what you are saying. It doesn't matter, continue to speak them aloud with as much conviction as you can muster. It's taken a long time to train your subconscious to use negative self talk. If you will persevere with speaking your affirmations aloud, firmly and confidently, you will be amazed at how quickly you can turn your thoughts around.

The Last Weight-loss Program You Will Ever Need

You didn't hop on a bicycle the first time and just take off down the street. It took practice to train your body to balance on those two wheels. This will take some practice as well. Continue to repeat your affirmations aloud, several times a day for the next 30 days and you will be amazed at how much you change your thinking and attitude.

Let's investigate how words affect you in your everyday life. Take a trip down memory lane and recall some real life experiences that made you happy, proud, successful or any combination of the three.

Spend some time recalling how you felt. Maybe you won a spelling bee as a child, or hit a home run. Who was there? This will help you remember that you had those feelings once and you can achieve them again. What words did others use while you were experiencing those feelings of joy and happiness.

Recall those words and put them to work in your daily conversations. They are words that are already proven to have a positive affect on your well being. Recalling and including them in your day will trigger those feelings again because your subconscious already has an association with those words and their results.

Above all, take action. If you have become a slave of procrastination decide to rid your life of it once and for all. Yes, you can create affirmations to help you there as well. "I have the attitude and skills to take action today." "I am winning in my life by turning my attitude into action."

Do nothing and nothing gets done. Do something and many things are placed in motion. Regardless of what you are doing in life, you need to take action. Do something every day to put your plan in motion.

How is your attitude? What are your first thoughts when you awake in the morning? You've got quite a lot to choose from. Do you begin the day by dragging out of bed bemoaning the fact that you have to get to work? Or, do you embrace the morning as another great opportunity to do great things?

Put the universal law of reciprocity to work in your life every single day. Did you know that as much as ninety nine percent of our conversation is negative? There are some folks who can hardly wait to get their mouths open so they can "one up" another persons current negative situation.

Hmmm, think back to that self talk. If what you hear every day is negative, it's no wonder your self talk brings you down and prevents you from being, doing and having everything you desire. Try this exercise. Make a decision today, right now, from this moment to spend the rest of the day contributing to conversation in a positive way.

Impossible, you say? Not so. Say that somebody complains about another rainy day. Your response might be, "yes, isn't it great, see that beautiful rainbow!" Try and create the habit of saying something positive to everyone.

If you are learning to say something positive to everybody about everything every time, you are disciplining your subconscious positive results in everything that happens to you.

TAKE ACTION

The Last Weight-loss Program You Will Ever Need

Before we can begin, we need to grasp an understanding of the problem.

More and more people are becoming overweight. The primary cause is that we eat more and exercise less. There is no doubt that the more advances we make that enhance our lifestyle the heavier we become.

Wait a minute! What about all those low-fat foods that we eat now? How come I reduced fat in my diet but I'm still gaining weight?

It's a simple answer. A few years ago we all became aware of the detrimental effects of fat in our diet. What did we do? We began to concentrate on lowering cholesterol and taking fat out of our diets.

This is a good thing. However, The National Center for Health Statistics studied eating habits of 8,260 adult American between 1988 and 1991. Their research showed that Americans had significantly reduced their fat intake but still packed on the pounds.

How can this happen? There is no mystery. In the process of counting fat grams, we stopped counting calories! Many of us bought in to the theory that if it's "low-fat" it won't make us fat.

WRONG!

You can't forget about counting calories. If you eat more calories than you need the body will store them as fat. It doesn't matter whether the calories are from fat or carbohydrates.

One school of thought believes that eating small amounts of fat can actually keep you from over indulging on total calories. The theory is that dietary fat causes our bodies to produce a hormone that tells the intestines to slow down the emptying process. You feel full and therefore are less likely to overeat.

Adding a little peanut butter to your rice cake may satisfy your hunger for a longer period of time, thus preventing you from eating more than you need.

Here's more news that is surprising. Tufts University scientists put 11 middle aged men and women volunteers on a variety of average, reduced and low-fat diets.

The results? Extremely low-fat diets which provided only 15 percent fat from calories (this is a diet near impossible in real life) did have a positive effect on blood cholesterol and triglyceride levels.

However, a reduced-fat diet (much more realistic)only affected those levels if accompanied by weight loss.

In fact, they concluded, cutting fat without losing weight actually increased triglyceride levels and decreased high density lipoproteins (HDLs), the "good" cholesterol that helps protect again heart disease.

We can deduce, therefore, while excess fat isn't healthy, it fat is also not necessarily a bad thing. Without some fat in our diet, the body won't make nerve cells and hormones or absorb some of the fat soluble vitamins.

Okay, so how can you determine your ideal weight? Just how much fat and how many calories should you consume to reach and maintain a healthy weight?

One answer won't work for everybody. So you need to do some figuring to determine how much fat and how many calories you can have. First, you need to determine your ideal weight. Here is a simple method to determine what that weight should be:

For Women

The ideal weight for a woman who is exactly 5 feet tall is 100 pounds. For every additional inch above 5 feet, add five pounds. If you are shorter than 5 feet tall, subtract five pounds for every inch you measure below 5 feet.

Next, determine whether you have a small, medium or large frame. Using a measuring tape, measure your wrist. If your wrist measures exactly 6 inches, you have a medium frame and the weight number you calculated above, does not need to be adjusted. If your wrist measures less than 6 inches, subtract 10 percent from your ideal weight. If your wrist measures more than 6 inches, add 10 percent to your ideal weight.

For Men

The ideal weight for a man who is exactly 5 feet tall is 106 pounds. For every additional inch above 5 feet, add 6 pounds. To determine whether you have a small, medium or large frame, measure your wrist. If your wrist measures exactly 7 inches, you have a medium frame and you do not need to adjust your ideal weight. If your wrist is smaller than 7 inches, you have a small frame and should subtract 10 percent from your ideal weight. If your wrist is larger than 7 inches, you have a small frame and should add 10 percent to your ideal weight.

Okay, now that you know what your ideal body weight should be, let's take a look at how many calories your body needs each day. Before we do this however, you need to take into account your level of activity.

If you are totally inactive and usually get no exercise, multiply your adjusted ideal weight by 11. If you get regular exercise two or three times a week, multiply your adjusted ideal weight by 13. If you get regular exercise four to five times a week, multiple your adjusted ideal weight by 15. And finally, if you get regular exercise six to seven times a week, multiply your adjusted ideal weight by 18.

Now that you know your ideal weight and how many calories you need each day you can easily figure out how much fat you can eat. Most nutritionists recommend that you limit daily intake of fat to 30 percent of your total calories. However, if you want to lose weight or have a history of heart disease or cancer, limit your daily fat intake to 20 percent of your total calories.

Let's take a look at a real life example. If Jane is a 5 foot 4 inch woman with a medium frame her ideal weight is 120 pounds. Jane is trying to lose weight so she need to keep her fat calories down to about 20 percent.

Jane is exercising two to three times a week so we can multiply her ideal weight by the number that matches her activity level, which is 13. Now we know that Jane need 1,560 calories each day.

If we take 20 percent of 1,560 (1,560 multiplied by .20) we get 312. Next, translate fat calories into fat grams (this will make it easier for you to read food labels). One gram of fat equals 9 calories. So if we divide 312 by 9 we know that Jane can eat abut 35 grams of fat per day.

Because Jane is over weight and trying to lose, her ideal weight and current weight do not match up. Jane needs to adjust her total calorie consumption. In order for her to lose one pound, she needs to eliminate 3,500 calories.

One simple solution is to lose a pound a week. That's a worthy, healthy goal and we'll explore methods that will help you achieve that goal in the upcoming segments.

Diet

Avoid "fad" diets. If you don't believe me, ask your doctor about these: negative calorie diets, extremely low calorie diets, low carb diets, and any other type of "fad" diet that is unbalanced.

Changing diet should be a matter of healthier life style. Learn all you can about different foods and nutrition. The more you know the easier it is to implement healthy nutrition in your diet.

∧∧

THE TIPS AND TRIGGERS START NOW!

>>>

1. Substitute fruit purees for butter or margarine. They are easy to prepare in a food processor and will significantly reduce calories and fat.
2. Cheese is good for you, but the fat is not. Try this: Zap cheese in the microwave and drain off grease.

3. Exercising before you eat just makes you hungrier. Exercise AFTER eating when the body has to work harder to digest food.

4. Don't eat while watching television. You can become so engrossed in your program that YOU don't realize how much you are eating.

5. Too many people skip breakfast. Eat in the morning when the body burns more calories. Breakfast is very important.

6. Water mixed with fructose suppresses appetite better than glucose with water or diet drinks. Drink a glass of orange juice one half to one hour before a meal.

7. Avoid fatty additives. Use olive, corn or canola oil when cooking.

8. Switch from whole to skim milk. All the nutrients are there without the fat. Okay, at least cut back to low fat!

9. Limit yourself to just four egg yolks a week.

10. Trim all fat from meats before cooking. You'll be amazed at how much you reduce your fat intake if you take this one small step.

11. Eliminate fried foods. Do we need to say why?

12. Cream sauces are loaded with fat. Use tomato based sauces instead of cream.

13. Use lemon juice or low sodium soy sauce for flavor.

14. Don't skip meals. When you do, you eat more at your next meal and usually eat the wrong foods.

15. Read labels – check fat, sugar and carb content.

16. Stop buying on impulse. Never shop for groceries without a list.

17. Avoid shopping when you are hungry – eat first!

18. Shop for groceries once a week and only buy from your prepared list.

19. Head directly to the fruit and vegetable aisles when you enter the grocery store. Fill up your basket in these aisles and you'll be less likely to buy binge food.

20. If you have a local "farmers market" where you can buy your fruits and veggies off the truck, by all means do so. They'll be fresher and tastier.

21. Make sure you buy everything you need for your weekly meal planning. Returning to the grocery store numerous times increases the risk of buying what you shouldn't. The grocery stores know their business very well and present items that are hard to resist.

22. Vary your foods – introduce something new each week. Menu planning can become boring when you eat the same things. That boredom translates into over eating. Try new healthy recipes each week.

23. Stay away from processed foods as much as possible. Yes, they are very convenient. They are also loaded with fat and/or sugar, not to mention the chemicals.

24. The ads are sooo compelling. Cut fast food from your diet!

25. Eat more fish but avoid breading or batters. Fish oil is good for you.

26. Eat more vegetables. Try mixing and matching fresh vegetables for variety.

27. Steam your veggies instead of boiling them. They'll taste better and you'll retain more of their nutritional value.

28. Use fat free or low fat salad dressings or make your own using lemon juice,

spices and a tiny amount of olive oil.

29. Exchange water for soft drinks – yes, even diet drinks!

30. Slim down with casseroles – just use lean meat and veggies.

31. Go ahead and snack, just snack on good stuff, like raisins, nuts veggies and dried fruit.

32. Never eat while you are standing.

33. Don't sample when you are cooking. A taste here, a little bite there and before you know it you've eaten an entire portions without sitting down at the table!

34. Don't give up potatoes. A baked potato has 0 grams of fat and only 160 calories. Just don't eat fries that weigh in at 13 fat grams and 480 calories!

35. Stay away from pastries. They are loaded with fat not to mention that they are also loaded with sugar.

36. Eat more salads but don't let salad become boring. Add different ingredients. Throw in a few raisins or canned beans and vary your dressings. Leave out the mayo!

37. Limit your intake of meat to just two or three meat choices per week and select more "white" meats than red.

38. You don't have to give up dessert, just rearrange it. Try mixing fresh fruits with low fat yogurt. Strawberries with banana yogurt are delicious!

39. Add nuts to your yogurt and salads. Chopped nuts make a great alternative to "breaded" style garnishes like croutons.

40. Replace white bread with whole grain bread. If you can find bread that still

contains the "wheat germ," buy it!

41. When baking, applesauce makes a great substitute for shortening.

42. Prepare foods in different ways. Instead of traditional frying, try stir-fry and use a low fat spray or non-stick pan.

43. Reduce portions at meal time. We live in a "jumbo size" world. There's no reason why the portions we consumer need to be super sized as well.

44. Measure portions one time to get an idea of what a portion of any given food should be. Do it once for each food that you commonly eat. Eventually, you will be able to "eyeball" a proper serving.

45. Keep a food diary of everything you eat. This is the first step to acquiring a new, healthier life style.

46. Take 5 meals, but in smaller portions. This regiment will help to stabilize your metabolism.

47. Specific food combinations can help to burn calories by enhancing your metabolism. Eat carbs that are rich in fiber. They take longer to digest and you will feel "fuller" for longer periods of time.

48. Use fresh or frozen fruits and vegetables. Canned veggies are okay in a pinch, but generally include more salt than you need. By the time they are canned and processed, they have lost much of their nutritive value.

49. Eat more yogurt. Yogurt is a protein as well as a carbohydrate therefore giving you the small amount of energy needed to burn the protein.

50. Add more tuna to your diet. You can grill it, broil it, steam it and poach it, all without any added fat.

51. Try different varieties of beans rather than sticking to the same old type you are accustomed to. Beans are a great source of energy, protein and fiber.

52. Beware of misleading claims. Reduced fat merely means that the item has 25% less fat. Use common sense. If something "normally" contains 300 fat grams, then reduced fat means it still has over 200 grams of fat!

53. Salads to avoid are tuna, chicken and egg. It isn't the meat or egg that's the problem. It's the mayonnaise. Try making them with plain yogurt and spices to dress it up and you'll have a healthy combination.

54. If you absolutely must have your fatty salad dressing, try this. Have the dressing on the side and dip your fork into the dressing before you spear the salad ingredient. You'll have your taste but without dredging your salad in fat.

55. Love avocado? Go ahead and indulge a quarter cup but don't mix it with sour cream!

56. Roasted, flavored almonds make a great snack.

57. Make your own potato chips. It's simple. Thinly slice a large baking potato and place in a single layer on a cookie sheet sprayed with low fat aerosol spray. Spray the slices lightly as well. Sprinkle with paprika and any other spice of your choosing. Bake in a 400 degree oven for thirty minutes making sure to turn once. 'Voila! Your own home baked potato chips and a great snack.

58. Switch from cream of wheat cereal to oatmeal. The whole grain in oatmeal is much better for you and won't leave you hungry an hour later like the cream of wheat.

59. If you plan on eating out at a buffet, eat something before you go. Don't skip a meal and plan on chowing down at the buffet.

60. Grab a table as far from the buffet as possible. You'll lessen the temptation to graze or go back for seconds.

61. Go through the buffet line one time only.

62. Load up at the salad bar. Gelatin or plan green salads should be abundant.

63. Pile on the grilled food looking for baked roasted or grilled entrees like fish or lean roast beef.

64. Avoid the breaded fish or fried chicken.

65. Select soups that you can see through. If you can see through them, they are broths with less fat and calories.

66. Eat slowly. Savor each bite. Take your time and enjoy eating. If you eat too fast, your stomach will be full long before the message to stop chowing down reaches your brain.

67. Ask yourself if you really tasted and enjoyed that last bite of food. If your answer is no, it's time to slow down.

68. To help downsize your portions, use a smaller plate. Instead of a dinner plate, use a salad plate for your entire meal.

69. When eating in a restaurant ask for a child's portion or ask to have the entrée split and have the second half packaged as takeout.

70. As an assist to making certain you are getting the right nutrition from your vegetables, alternate the colors from day to day. One day eat fresh yellow and orange vegetables like squash, pumpkin, and carrots then switch to

green the next day, like spinach, or dark leafy lettuces.

71. Pass up peanuts for snacking. Two ounces of salted peanuts has 328 calories. Nibble on pretzels instead. 20 of the small ones have as little as 80 calories and most are fat free.

72. Skip fried shrimp. A three ounce serving has 206 calories while the same size boiled is only 84 calories.

73. If you love pie, stick with the fruit pies. Pumpkin and other fruit pies are lower in calories. Pecan pie has about 430 calories while the same slice of pumpkin pie is only 240. You can drop another 100 calories if you don't eat the crust!

74. Try Canadian bacon instead of regular bacon. One ounce of regular bacon is about four medium cooked slices and carries 163 calories. A one ounce slice of Canadian bacon is much leaner and only has about 57 calories.

75. Avoid the high fat temptations when dining out. Call ahead. Many high quality restaurants will accommodate your needs if you give them sufficient time beforehand. Explain that you are on a low fat diet and ask if they can prepare your food without frying.

76. If you frequent a specific restaurant, ask to take a menu home so you can study what they offer and learn how to plan your meals out.

77. Avoid fast food restaurants. Most of their food is 40 to 50 percent fat. Many are finally wising up, however, and you can get salads, plain hamburgers or grilled chicken. You can also ask for the restaurant's nutritional information. Many now offer that.

78. Stay away from the appetizers unless you request crackers, pretzels or fresh vegetables like carrots or celery with a honey-mustard dressing (not ranch).

79. Put your waiter through his or her paces. Ask lots of questions and don't stop until you are satisfied. How is the fish grilled? If it is in butter, ask for it dry. If a fried entrée is offered on the menu, ask if the chef can bake it, broil it, grill it or steam it to cut down on the fat. Make sure they follow up. It's your meal and your money paying for it and within reason you should be able to get it the way you want it.

80. If a restaurant won't split a portion in half for you, preparing half of it "to go," request a doggie bag or box be delivered with your meal and split it yourself immediately before you begin to eat.

81. You can also carry a "survival kit." Use a small plastic sandwich bag and carry packets of low fat dressings, herbal teas, spices or other essentials that may not be readily available at a restaurant.

82. Split a meal with a friend. Order soup or salad a' la carte with one entrée and ask the waiter for an extra plate. It will save you money AND reduce the fat in each meal.

83. Visit pizzerias that offer salads and pizza by the slice. Don't order pizza with meat. Stick with vegetable toppings and, if possible, a wheat crust. Some pizza places do offer that option.

84. Eliminate tartar sauce. If you order a fish fillet sandwich ask that the tartar sauce be left off the bun.

85. Bake with cocoa instead of chocolate. For each ounce of unsweetened

chocolate called for in a recipe, substitute 3 tablespoons of unsweetened cocoa powder.

86. Use evaporated skim milk for sauces and soups. It has the texture and the flavor of cream but without the fat. Each cup contains 80 grams less of fat and 600 few calories than heavy cream.

87. Plain nonfat or low fat yogurt is a great replacement for sour cream. Use it to make salad dressings. It's also good as an add on to breakfast cereals and desserts.

88. Low fat foods may seem less flavorful when you first try them because fat adds flavor to some foods and you are used to that. Add zip with lots of herbs and spices like basil, garlic, ginger, onion powder tarragon and oregano. Vary the spices and come up with your own combinations.

89. Yogurt can help you lose weight while protecting muscle. A recent study of overweight people who at three servings of yogurt daily for 12 weeks lost 22% more weight, 61% more body fat and 81%more abdominal fat than people who ate a similar number of calories but no dairy products.

90. Spicy foods curb appetite as evidenced in a recent study. People who ate a sauce containing *capsaicin* (the compound that makes hot pepper spicy), consumed an average of 200 fewer calories over the next three hours than those who didn't eat the sauce. Consider eating more spicy foods.

91. A 12 ounce cola has 150 calories, two tablespoons of full fat salad dressing 150, a glazed doughnut 250 and a four ounce bagel, 300. Just eliminating these items will help you to lose weight.

92. Another recent study shows that calcium from diary foods is more effective for weight loss than supplements. Why? Food is a complex mixture of known and unknown components. There is a cooperation among the components that can't be reproduced in a nutritional supplement. Dairy contains calcium and a host of other biologically active components including the amino acid leucine. Recent research reveals that leucine may increase the ability of muscle to use fat. Have low-fat or skim milk before a meal.

   Studies show that getting a liquid form f dairy before eating helps you feel fuller sooner at that meal and eat less at the next meal. If you are lactose intolerant, try yogurt with live culture (it has very little lactose) or take a lactose supplement when consuming dairy.

93. Eat fish at least twice a week. The omega 3 fatty acids in fish have been shown to reduce heart attack and stroke risk in addition to helping you maintain a nutritional diet.

94. Sometimes you can go with fast food. Burger Kings Bl Veggie Burger with reduced fat mayonnaise contains 340 calories and 2 grams of saturated fat. It's better than just about any burger at any other food chain.

95. McDonald's Fruit and Yogurt Parfait is low fat vanilla yogurt layered with berries and topped with granola. It's a nutrient rich bargain at only 380 calories.

96. Subway's 7 subs with 6 grams of fat or less include ham, roast beef, chicken and turkey and range from 200 to 300 calories for a six inch sub.

97. Wendy's Mandarin Chicken Garden Sensation Salad is a creative salad

alternative of mixed greens, chicken and mandarin orange sections, roasted almonds and a half packet of Oriental sesame dressing is a great alternative at just 470 calories.

98. A veggie sandwich may not always be the ideal choice. The two ounces of cheese added to these popular lunchtime meals contain three quarters of a full day's allowance for saturated fat. Tuna salad (because of the mayonnaise), has 720 calories and chicken salad is 550 calories. Stick with turkey, roast beef, chick breast or veggie sandwich without the cheese.

99. All salads are not created equal. A taco salad is served in a fried taco shell filled with ground beef, cheese, sour cream and guacamole. It contains 1,100 calories a full day's quota of saturated fat!

100. Not only is a single order of Fettucine Alfredo an artery clogger, it also weighs in at a whopping 1,500 calories! When eating Italian food, opt for pasta topped with marinara or meat sauce (skip the meatballs), red or white clam sauce or chicken Marcala.

EXERCISE

Well, you knew it was coming, didn't you? We've discussed at least 100 ways to adjust your eating habits. Some of the tips we covered will help your metabolism burn extra calories, but the bottom line is that you still need to burn more calories than you consume if you wish to lose those extra pounds.

The dawn of the Information Age has given us more labor saving devices than any other period in history. Along with this knowledge we have settled into a more sedentary lifestyle.

The Last Weight-loss Program You Will Ever Need

Taking a little trip back in time can really open our eyes. A typical day for your great grandmother began long before the sunrise. She was usually the first to awaken so she could have a hearty breakfast on the table for the rest of the family.

She would probably stoke her range with wood brought in the previous evening. Unless one of the children were old enough to be charged with the task, she would put on her coat, scarf and gloves and trek out to the barn to milk the cow, stopping on her way back to gather eggs from the chicken coop, home-cured ham and sausage from the smoke house, cheese (that she had made herself) butter (that she churned) and potatoes from the cold storage cellar.

Returning to her kitchen with her collection in tow, she would prepare a breakfast that most likely consisted of ham, sausage and eggs fried in lard she had rendered, biscuits, gravy made from the leavings in the frying pan, flapjacks, whole milk and strong coffee.

That picture can pretty much turn your veins to instant concrete!

Bear in mind that after her pre-dawn preparations she would spend the remainder of her day, sweeping, dusting, polishing, scrubbing clothing using hot water that she boils herself, hanging the laundry out to dry, tending her vegetable garden and often toiling in the fields with the men.

The comparison between your great grandparents is not so much what they ate, as how they used the calories they consumed. Life was hard. Normal physical activity usually burned off the calories they consumed. They worked hard and ate hearty and, yes they did have a shorter life expectancy.

The Last Weight-loss Program You Will Ever Need

Today we eat foods that are processed and contain more fat and chemicals than nutrition. To top it off, we also live sedentary lives. Unlike grandma's hearty breakfast we are more likely to grab a cup of coffee on the run. We rush to an office, only to spend the next 8 hours sitting in front of a computer screen, just as you are doing now.

Getting a handle on your diet is just the first step toward losing weight and living a healthier lifestyle. In order to tame the weight loss beast, you MUST change your physical habits as well as your eating habits.

You don't necessarily have to exert yourself as if you were training for the Olympics, but you definitely need to learn how to burn off more calories than you consume. Once you have accomplished that, you can step in to a regimen to maintain your ideal weight.

Before you begin a fitness/exercise program, you need to know what you want to accomplish. Use the information in the chapter on "Where To Begin" to determine your ideal weight. Once you have your plan firmly in place (we will discuss this further in the next chapter) you can begin to incorporate the following tips.

101.   Always warm up before beginning your exercise activity using smooth and fluid movement. The purpose of the warm up is to minimize discomfort and prevent injury and loosen up your muscles for the exercise to come.

102.   Begin with a couple of deep breaths, inhaling through the nose and exhaling from your mouth.

103.   When you plan to walk or run, do just a few hundred yards at a slower walk or a gentler jog.

104.   Use the cool down routine in the reverse of the warm-up, gently slowing down. This will enable your breathing and heart rate to return to normal.

105.   Learn to listen to your body and differentiate between *good* pain and *bad* pain.

106.   Never exercise on a full or empty stomach.

107.   Drink plenty of water to reduce the chance of dehydration. Experts usually recommend 16 ounces either one or two hours before exercising.

108.   Always use stretching routines. These are not just for jocks and fitness gurus but should be used by everyone. The older you are, the more important this becomes as you can help retain flexibility and good range of movement for all your daily activities.

109.   When warming up and stretching, use the movements for five to ten minutes. This will help to loosen your muscles.

110.   Do not bounce when warming up with stretching as you can cause tears in your muscle fibers.

111.   To increase your flexibility, hold each stretch for fifteen to twenty seconds or longer.

112.   Be sure you stretch lightly during warm up to prevent stretch reflex. This is caused by over using a cold muscle.

113.   Breathe slowly and evenly throughout your warm up.

114.   If you have a tendency to become stiff, take a hot shower or bath

before beginning your warm up.

115.   Breathing is extremely important when exercising as your body need to process oxygen that will transfer from your lungs through the bloodstream to the muscles that are being worked. Normal breathing is shallow meaning that the air is not reaching deep into the lungs. This can tighten neck muscles which can cause stiffness and pain in the neck, shoulder upper back and chest.

116.   Always inhale before you lift, exhale as you lift and inhale as you lower the weight for maximum benefit.

117.   Turn every day activity into exercise. Try balancing on one foot without support while putting on your shoes and socks.

118.   Forget about the elevator and use the stairs.

119.   Take the stairs two at a time.

120.   Instead of shoving your chair, lift it bending your knees and keeping your back straight.

121.   Hide your remote control and get up and down to change the channels.

122.   Walk your dog and keep pace.

123.   Take a Frisbee along and play in the park with your dog.

124.   Park in the furthest parking space.

125.   Instead of sitting in the stands while watching your kids play at a ballgame, try pacing the field instead.

126.   Clean your house (changing bedding is great exercise!).

127. Take a brisk ten minute walk each morning, afternoon and evening.

128. Plant a vegetable garden. You'll have all that terrific food to eat and exercise in the process!

129. Learn how to snorkel.

130. Learn a new dance.

131. Join a gym.

132. Join a lunch hour aerobic class.

133. When exercising, use a multi-purpose squat to improve strength in the lower body. This will strengthen all of the major muscles of the lower body including hamstrings, quadriceps, calves and gluteals.

134. Use balance training exercises to help in performing daily living and activities. Try a one-legged balance exercise by standing on one leg for 10 to 15 seconds, switching legs and repeating the process for three to five sets.

135. Jump in place with feet together. Alternate between touching the left and right heel in between jumps with both feet.

136. Target the triceps with a bench dip. Seated on a bench, grasp the front edge with your hands shoulder-width apart. With your heels on the florr, extend your legs straight out from your body. Move forward until your hips are off the bench. Lower the hips slowly toward the floor then press up to a full extension of your arm without locking your elbows.

137. Try a bent over row to target the latissimus dorsi, teres major, posterior deltoid, trapezius, rhomboids and biceps. While standing, begin with your feet should width apart. Bend the knee and flex forward at the hips. Tilting

the pelvis slightly forward, engage the abdominals and extend the upper spine to add additional support. Hold a weight or bar beneath the shoulders with your hands approximately should width apart. Flex your elbows and lift your hands toward the sides of your body. Pause and slowly lower your hand back to the starting position. Be sure to keep your shoulders stationary.

138.   A simple shoulder shrug can help to strengthen your back. Stand erect with dumbbells or other weight in each hand. Lift your shoulders toward your head by elevating your shoulders and slightly retract and roll them back. Pause for a moment then return to the starting position. Make certain that you do not rock or use your legs and keep your knees slightly bent. A variation on this exercise is to do one shoulder at a time.

139.   Another exercise to strengthen the back is a scapular retraction. Begin with your feet shoulder width apart and your pelvis tilted and slightly forward. Engage your abbdominals so you can maintain neutral spine. Flex forward and hold dumbbells extended down and away from the body. Flex the shoulder blades together, pausing then slowly returning to the start position. Avoid bending your elbows and vary the exercise by using a single arm at a time.

140.   Remember to keep it slow. Perform all exercises slowly. Spend two to five seconds in the lifting phase of an exercise and four to six seconds in the lowering part. If you move too quickly, you won't get the muscle strengthening benefit of the exercise and you could hurt yourself.

141.   Work up to the point where you can do three sets of each exercise, with five to 15 repetitions of the exercise in each set. Don't rest within the sets,

you can rest briefly between each set. As the work becomes easier ad weights or increase the number of repetitions you do.

142.   Bicycling gives a great whole body exercise. Begin with short jaunts around your neighborhood. Each day widen your travels until you are able to bicycle for at least a mile.

143.   Exercise should give you additional energy. If you are excessively exhausted after exercising you have overdone it.

144.   Again, listen to your body. If you experience a feeling of nausea or faintness, your efforts may be too intense for your body or you aren't spending enough time on your cool down process.

145.   Your rate of breathing will increase while exercising but you should still be able to carry on a conversation. If you can't talk and walk or talk and lift at the same time, your pace is probably too intense. Cut back and lighten your weight load.

146.   While you may experience some next day soreness when you begin, exercise isn't supposed to hurt or leave you feeling stiff. Devote more time to warm up and cool down exercises as your body adjusts.

147.   Being overweight, your knees may not be strong enough to support you. If you experience pain, then shorten (or eliminate) your walks, jogs or bicycling and concentrate on strength building sessions to build up your muscles and tendons.

148.   If you have been sedentary, you may experience lower back pain when you first begin to exercise. This is because your hamstring muscles have

shortened. When you walk or exercise the shortened hamstrings pull on the buttock muscles which in turn will grab your lower back muscles. If your abdominal muscles are not strong enough to assist in supporting your lower back, you will definitely feel it. To get rid of the pain, include abdominal strengthening exercises with your warm up and cool down.

149.   If you get a headache, cramps or heart palpitations, or feel dizzy, faint or cool while exercising, consult your physician.

150.   If you have an infection such as bronchitis, put off exercise until all is normal again.

151.   If you just have a cold or the flu, wait until all symptoms such as fever, have been gone for two days before you exercise again.

152.   Walking is the aerobic exercise of preference if you are over 60. This is because when you walk, the pressure on your joints never rises about 1.5 times your body weight. Jogging, dance or step aerobics can put as much as four times your weight or more on your bones. This is wonderful for younger people, but can put too much strain on the more brittle bones of the elderly.

153.   Start your walking exercise by timing yourself. You don't want to become too tried to make it back home. Check your watch when you begin, and walk around one block over and over until you get a little tired. Check your watch to see how long you have walked. That's the length that your walks should be for the first week or two. If you get tired on the way home, stop, rest then walk some more…

✦ **Don't forget, now is a good time to work on your VISUALIZATION…Remember, the movie format. Go on do it!**

154.   Maintain the same level of exertion for your entire walk. You will be asking your heart to work hard (but not too hard) for your entire session. Your hearts gets the biggest benefit from a sustained workout. If you come to a hill, slow your pace to maintain the same level of exertion that you had on ground level.

155.   If the temperature is hot or humid your workout will seem harder. Adjust the speed and intensity so that you stay at the appropriate exertion level.

156.   If the temperature soars over 95°F with 80% humidity, limit outside exercise to no more than 30 to 45 minutes.

157.   Establish a rhythm to your exercise routine. Using music can help you to do this. The rhythm helps you perform each repetition within a set with the same gusto!

158.   Be kind to your feet. Exercise in shoes that were designed for the job or you are giving an open invitation to aches, pains and even stress fractures in your feet and legs.

159.   Pick the right kind of shoe. Walking or running shoes absorb the shock of your stride. This is thanks to a slightly elevated heel that also helps to prevent injuries to the leg muscles and tendons.

160.   Tennis and other types of athletic shoes absorb the impact of sideways movement and quick turns.

161.   Women who typically wear high heels should avoid flat tennis type shoes because the sudden shift in foot position could cause strain.

162.   Buy new shoes often. They may last for years, but looks are deceiving. They will lose their shock absorption within just a few months. If you walk fewer than 25 miles a week a new pair is in order every four to six months. If you walk more than 25 miles a week, they should be replaced every two to three months.

163.   Examine the patterns in your existing shoes and/or take them along when shopping for new ones. Your wear patterns might help the salesperson pick out the best pair for your feet.

164.   To get the best fit wear or bring along the same kind of socks that you will be exercising in. Shop in the afternoon in case your feet swell during the day.

165.   After your warm up, exercise for more than 30 minutes per session if you want to lose weight. Otherwise, three 10 minutes sessions per day will protect against disease and a healthier lifestyle.

166.   Wear loose fitting clothing that breathes well. You can use layers of clothing to stay warm and dispel perspiration and heat.

167.   Avoid drinking coffee, alcohol or other diuretics before or while you exercise.

168.   If you are a morning person, exercise after you have been up and about for at least 10 minutes. While sleeping, sometimes fluids can pool throughout your body even in disks in the spinal column, ligaments and muscles.

If you get up and immediately begin to exercise, the accumulated fluids can cause major injury such as a herniated disk.

169.   Avoid exercise right after eating. Both your intestinal tract and your muscles will need extra blood to function. The conflicting needs of each system may leave you with cramps or a feeling of nausea or faintness. Give you body two hours to complete its digestive duties.

170.   If you have diabetes, avoid injecting insulin into a muscle that will soon be used for exercise. Working muscles process insulin differently than nonworking muscles.

171.   Learn how much activity is required per hour to burn calories. For instance, one hour of bicycling at 6 miles per hour burns 240 calories; at 12 miles per hour, you will burn 410 calories. Jogging at 5.5 miles per hours burns 740 calories but at just 2 miles per hour more at 7 miles per hour you will burn 920 calories.

172.   Walking at just 2 mph, burns 240 calories; increase it to 3 mph and you are burning 320 calories and at 4.5 mph you are burning a whopping 440 calories! *Note that this is based on a healthy 150 pound woman. A lighter person burns fewer calories, a heavier person burns more.

173.   Walking need not be a chore. Visit your local museums and art galleries spending time browsing the exhibits. Not only will you add additional exercise with the walk, you'll improve your mind!

174.   Eating a handful of raisins (about 1 ounce) approximately 15 minutes before your workout can significantly lower free radical and the damage

they cause. **Raisins are rich in antioxidants.**

175.   In addition to your daily workout here is a simple exercise to do while sitting at your desk, driving or watching television. From a sitting position, sit up tall and pull your abdominal muscles in, lifting your chest and rib cage as you exhale. Hold for four to six seconds then release slowly as you inhale. Repeat eight to 12 times. If you do this while driving, adjust your rearview mirror so you can see out of it only when you are in the sitting tall position. This will remind you to maintain this posture.

176.   Here is a quick way to tone up your buttocks whenever or wherever (almost) you are standing. Squeeze the buttock muscles in both cheeks as tightly as you can, then hold the contraction for two seconds. Release for two seconds then repeat eight to 12 times.

177.   Need to strengthen your calves? Stand on a telephone book (the bigger the better) with your toes facing the book spine and your heels hanging over the edge opposite the spine. For better stability this exercise can also be done standing on a step while holding a railing or on a curb while holding a signpost for balance. Keeping your back straight, push up onto the balls of your feet while counting for two seconds, hold for another two seconds, then count for four seconds as you lower yourself back down. Tighten up your abdominals and buttocks to help stay balanced.

YOUR DESTINATION

I'd like to leave you with a few thoughts that may help you on your weight loss journey. At the beginning, we discussed how the words we speak are very powerful and how those words create an attitude.

How often have you used the term, "my weight?" You may have made the comments like these:

"when I lose my weight. . . ."

"My weight doesn't let me. . ."

"I can't. . . .Because of my weight"

Do you see a common thread throughout these statements? Can you make an educated guess at how many times you have said one of them or something similar?

From our earlier discussion, you probably already noticed the "negative" affirmations . . .when. . .doesn't. . .can't. . . Read them again more carefully. Do you see the other critical factor in each statement?

Each of those statements re-affirm that you "own" your weight. Therefore, each time you make that comment not only are you re-affirming your current weight, you are pronouncing to the world that you are not willing to let go.

Using a personal pronoun is powerful stuff in and of itself because not only are you claiming ownership, you are training your subconscious mind to believe that you can't let go.

Starting today, right now, this very minute, make a conscious decision, that you no longer accept ownership of excess weight. You are not what you weigh. You are a unique human being and entitled to all the gifts that this life has to offer.

The Last Weight-loss Program You Will Ever Need

Now pull out pen and paper and begin your affirmations.

****

BOOK TWO-Secrets To Looking Younger!

SECRETS TO LOOKING AND FEELING YOUNGER

TABLE OF CONTENTS

The Last Weight-loss Program You Will Ever Need

INTRODUCTION

The truth is we begin the aging process just as soon as we pop out of the womb. Every day of our lives our bodies slough off and regenerate new cells. The speed at which that process takes place when we are children is vastly different as we get older.

For years explorers searched for the illusive "fountain of youth." Unfortunately, it does not exist or you wouldn't be reading this.

Every day you are bombarded daily with commercial messages that attempt to lure you into believing that the most recent miracle drug is just what you need to fight off the ravages of Mother Nature.

At times it seems as though there are more miracle methods than ever being flashed in front of your eyes each day. . .and there are. Ask any advertising executive and they will admit that there are more advertisements than ever touting everything designed to cash in on a huge market. What is that market? It's the aging Baby Boomers.

We are living longer as a whole. Singularly, that can be a curse or a blessing depending on your perspective. In this book we will explore low and no cost methods you can use to help in the anti-aging process.

Some of our material may be new and some serve as reminders of things we may have forgotten. We may not have had much say in how we arrived on this earth, but we can certainly determine how and when we will depart. Just

The Last Weight-loss Program You Will Ever Need

remember, YOU are in control.

LIFESTYLE

We have to discuss it. You've heard it before but it must be repeated. You ARE what you eat. There are over 13.5 million Americans alive today who have a history of heart attacks, angina or a combination of both. 50% of them are age 60 or older and 83% who die of heart attacks are 65 or more.

Today, many doctors rank fat intake right up there with smoking for leading cause of death. What can you do about? Plenty.

Fat – Americans love fat. We love fat so much that we eat the equivalent of 1 ½ cups of butter every week! Yes, that's correct. Walk to your refrigerator and pull out 6 sticks of butter and imagine them placed at different points in and out of your body. Pretty scary, isn't it? Excess fat intake is directly attributable to:

- Elevated cholesterol
- Elevated triglycerides
- High blood pressure
- Diabetes
- Excess weight.

Taking control of just this single area of your overall health will substantially reduce your chances of heart disease as well as reducing the risk of stroke. Stroke occurs when blood clots block arteries that supply blood to the brain.

French researchers examined 250 men and women age 60 to 70 and found that those who had fatty plaque narrowing the main artery out of the heart were 9 times more likely to have a stroke than those who did not have this buildup.

Cancer is another possible by-product of excess fat in the diet. In fact dietary fat is credited with playing a role in as much as 40% of cancers in men and 60% of cancers in women. Read meat is considered to be one of the biggest culprits, increasing the instance of colon, rectal and prostate cancer in men. For women the results are colon and possibly breast cancer. And, researchers are now beginning to believe it may play a role in lung cancer as well.

So why do we still eat it? Believe it or not, many of us just haven't gotten the word yet, especially those over 60. Even though the information about fat has been around for a long time, many people believe that fat is a necessary part of diet. Yes, it is true that dietary fat exists for a reason. It does provide us with the fatty acids we need to control our body temperature, give us healthy skin and hair and protect nerves and our vital organs.

The problem is that not all fats are created equal and many of us just don't understand the difference.

Monounsaturated fats such as olive and canola oils and polyunsaturated fats like corn and safflower oils are considered somewhat healthy when taken in moderation.

Saturated fats that we find predominantly in meat, eggs and dairy products are attributed with causing major health problems especially when consumed in large amounts.

Trans-fatty acids are another type of harmful fat. These are unsaturated fats that food manufacturers use to solidify certain foods like margarine and vegetable shortening. In addition to being harmful they have no dietary value at all.

It is unfortunate that a typical American meal does not consist of one type of fat or another but a combination of several so that when we eat we can consume a large amount of bad fat.

Switching to a low-fat style of eating mostly unsaturated fats you may very well quickly feel rejuvenated regardless of your age. No matter what your age or medical conditions might be, diabetes, high cholesterol, gout or heart disease a low-fat diet is the way to go.

Limit saturated fat to less than 10% of your daily calories and cut back on the fatty acids and the benefits will increase life expectancy.

Fiber – If there was one element of our diets that we would 'wish away' it might be fiber. Fiber is what is left over after our bodies have squeezed every bit of nutritive value from the foods we eat. Don't discount fiber, however. It is a very important part of a healthy diet.

Sadly, most older Americans get no more than 14.8 grams of fiber a day when you actually need 25 to 35 grams to protect against disease!

You can make up the difference by changing dietary habits and do it easily. Researchers have found an astounding 33% drop in cholesterol in some patients who did nothing more than increase fiber and reduce fat. And, there is research being conducted that indicates the perillyl alcohol contained in fiber shows promise of actually slowing down the growth of certain cancer tumors.

Before we take a look at how fiber can combat cancer, we need to explore the two different types of fiber – insoluble and soluble. Each type works differently to fight disease.

Insoluble fiber comes from a substance that forms in the cell walls of plants. The reason it is called insoluble is because your body does not break it down as it passes through the digestive system. It is what gives your stool its bulk helping it to move faster through your system. This is why certain foods that are high in soluble fiber like bran are said to be natures laxatives.

Grain products and vegetables have loads of fiber. While at first look it appears more as rabbit food than cancer fighting, studies show that insoluble fiber helps to fight colon cancer and researchers believe it also helps to fight breast, pancreatic and prostate cancers as well.

In Finland low rates of breast and colon cancer are linked directly to diets rich in cereals.

Certain parts of Africa where people consume lots of high fiber foods the incidence of intestinal disease is practically nil.

Let's take a look at how it works.

Insoluble fiber will soak up water as if it were a sponge thereby making stools bulkier. That excess bulk spreads out cancer causing components over a larger area preventing them from grouping together to do damage.

The Last Weight-loss Program You Will Ever Need

Fiber is the equivalent of a super highway through the intestines that gets things moving faster so there are fewer opportunities for any interaction between cells lining the colon and any cancerous agents.

Fiber works with the levels of acids in the intestines changing the way that certain bacteria do the job. The result is increased fermentation. Yes, it may cause gas but it also makes it harder for carcinogens to get in your body. It also plays a role in regulating the levels of intestinal bile acids that play a part in the beginning stages of colon cancer.

The "stuff" that causes breast, pancreatic and prostate cancers latch onto fiber like a magnet which means that those carcinogens are carried away with other body waste.

Researchers believe that insoluble fiber also contributes to reducing levels of harmful estrogen that can contribute to the beginning of breast cancer. Experiments appear to suggest that doubling fiber intake and reducing fat can reduce the tumor rate by 50%.

If you can imagine eating foods that can actually stop or slow the growth of tumors wouldn't you want to eat it? Well, you can.

Whether canned or dried, Beans in any form contain large amounts of fiber. Reduce the amount of gas by soaking them overnight in clean, clear water. Rinse again thoroughly before cooking.

Oat bran added to cereals or eaten as bread is a great source for additional fiber.

Try eating brown rice instead of white. Brown rice will supply 3.32 grams of fiber per cup while white rice contains only 0.74 grams per cup.

Whole grain bread products are a must. You can receive 3 grams or more of fiber per slice. Refined wheat loses fiber and removes trace minerals.

Read the labels in the grocery store, especially the fine print. The labels will tell you the fiber content of the food per serving. If the first three or four ingredients listed are grains it means that the product contains more grains than anything else.

Learn to balance the benefit of fiber versus other ingredients. If a granola bar has one or more grams of fiber it is only a good deal if the fat and calorie content are low. A snack bar with 100 calories, 2 grams of fat and a single gram of fiber is probably okay. But if the bar contains 300 calories and more fat that's way more than you need.

Introduce fiber in your diet one step at a time, gradually increasing and setting goals you can realistically attain. Storing easy to prepare foods in your pantry can help. Stock up on low-fat soups, canned beans and cereals that are all easy to prepare. Keep your freezer filled with vegetable that can be quickly steamed or zapped in your microwave.

Keep the liquid from canned beans. There's a lot of soluble fiber there that may just go down the drain. Save it to use in soups.

Don't peel fruits and vegetables. The skins of apples, pears, peaches and potatoes are rich in soluble fiber. Eating the white rind of oranges and the membrane in grapefruit also provide extra fiber.

Eat fruits and vegetable whole rather than as juices. You may get concentrated nutrients from the juices but you lose the fiber in the fruit. The 14 grams of fiber you get from eating six carrots outweighs the 2 grams in the juice you created with those 6 carrots.

Some people prefer taking a fiber supplement. There are many on the market, but be aware that most contain psyllium. While it is a source of fiber and a natural laxative it can interfere with certain medications you take. Be sure and check with your doctor.

Food – While we have discussed certain foods high in fiber, we haven't even scratched the surface of foods that can help you battle the aging process.

Plants. Nope, not the philodendron hanging in your kitchen window, but the treasure you find in the fruit and vegetable aisles of your supermarket. If there is one single piece of advice you can get from studying the aging process, consuming more fruits and vegetables are among the most important.

When you eat food made from plants, you are receiving the benefits of a small army marching off to combat the aging process. This army is comprised of agents known as phytochemicals. These are completely separate from the vitamins provided by the vegetable themselves but may be even more valuable.

Science used to believe that phytochemicals were absolutely useless. However as more experts delve into the study of plants they have found that they appear to help fight off cancer, heart disease and stroke even though they don't understand why. In fact over 200 studies conducted show that a diet high in fruits and veggies substantially cut the risk of cancer. That alone becomes increasingly important as you get older and the risk of disease increases.

Some of these phytochemicals are simple to detect. The bright orange color of carrots, sweet potatoes or yams are obvious. The pungent whiff of phytochemicals is apparent in garlic. However, most are undetectable.

The chemicals are there to actually protect the plant. It is believed that they evolved to protect plants from oxygen, wind, insects and weather. Remember that plants feed on carbon dioxide and oxygen is actually waste.

Without protection from the ultraviolet rays of a hot sun plants would shrivel and die. In the dirt where bulb plants grow, they are subjected to the hazards of bacteria and insects.

Edward Miller, Ph.D., professor of biomedical sciences in the Department of Biomedical Sciences at Baylor College of Dentistry in Houston states that, "We can save more than 150,000 lives a year, right now, with no treatments, no medical costs, no long-term recovery – if people would just eat the foods that protect them."

Worldwide studies have proven that phytochemicals protect against, but there is no one phytochemical or any other substance that you can take or eat for protection.

Eating plant foods does give you a lower risk for cancers that attack the lungs, bladder, cervix, mouth, larynx, throat, esophagus, stomach, pancreas, colon and rectum. Laboratory studies show that phytochemicals prevent cancer forming substances and defective cell that can turn into cancers, from gaining a foothold or spreading.

Phytochemicals also help to keep your heart healthy. The 60 to 80 age group that has a higher risk of heart disease than younger people do, can substantially reduce the risks by eating a diet rich in fruits and vegetables.

Plant foods also combat free radicals. Many phytochemicals do double duty as anti-oxidants. They neutralize the free radicals which are unstable molecules that damage or destroy healthy cells.

In addition to the free radicals that your body produces routinely, they also find their way into your environment through other means like cigarette smoke, pollutants, medications, pesticides as well as household cleaners.

They have also been linked to more than 60 medical problems and diseases. In addition to the obvious disease like heart disease, cancer and stroke, they can also manifest as premature aging, stiff joints, wrinkled skin, arthritis, diabetes and cirrhosis of the liver.

The study of phytochemicals in plants is a relatively new field, but here is a list of those that appear to provide the most protection:

Organosulfur compounds. These are foods that we recognize mostly by their pungent odor and flavor. Garlic, onions, leeks, chives and shallots are organosulfur compounds. You can also find these compounds in vegetables like broccoli, cabbage and cauliflower.

Foods that are rich in organosulfur are sometimes referred to by some members of the medical community as dietary anti-carcinogens. They help the body block and eliminate cancer causing agents before they do their damage. They are also instrumental in fighting heart disease and stroke.

The best methods to derive the most benefit from organosulfur compounds is to eat them raw or lightly cooked. Puree vegetables into a healthy soup and be sure to add garlic and onion.

Isothiocyanates are plant chemicals found in leafy green vegetable like watercress, arugula, cabbage, brussel sprouts, Chinese cabbage, broccoli and cauliflower. These compounds help rid the body of cancer causing substances and actually act to remove the trash. Isothicyanates make it difficult for cancer causing substances to target the DNA of healthy cells and in laboratory experiments have actually kept tumors from forming.

The most benefit you can receive from isothiocyanates in your food is to eat some of the vegetables raw. The compounds are released when chopped and chewed. Eat them as fresh as possible and eat plenty of them.

Indoles go with isothiocyanates like salt and pepper complement one another. Indoles protect against breast cancer in women and prostate cancer in men. Indoles stop the growth of small virus caused tumors. You can best benefit from indoles by eating the equivalent of a quarter head of cabbage a day or an equal amount of broccoli, Brussels sprouts or cauliflower.

Isoflavones are a group of plant estrogens that are found in soy products. To help increase your soy consumption, try tofu. It is far less bland when it absorbs the taste of spices and other foods that are cooked with it. Try more Asian recipes or drinking soy milk. When you are baking trade off 25% of your regular flour for soy flour. You'll get all the benefit with little or no difference in the recipe.

Lignans. Little is known about lignans as it is a newer area for research.

The Last Weight-loss Program You Will Ever Need

What is known, however, is that lignans seem to prevent breast cancer at lest in the laboratory. As antioxidants they may help prevent damage from LDL cholesterol which, as we know, lays the groundwork for heart disease.

Add lignans to your diet by including flax. Some baking companies add a trace amount of flax or linseed to add a slightly nutty flavor. You can find flax in health food stores, but use it very sparingly as adding it to your diet too quickly can cause intestinal distress.

Carotenoids are evidenced in the bright red, orange and yellow pigments displayed in some plants like carrots, tomatoes, sweet potatoes, cantaloupe, winter squash, parsley, green peas, pink grapefruit, swiss chard, spinach, beet greens, pumpkin, watermelon, broccoli, mangoes, oranges, papaya and tangerines. You will also find them in okra, red peppers leafy green vegetable and even in fish liver oil.

Diets rich in carotenoids fight disease and in one study a high carotenoid diet actually helped reduce the risk of lung cancer in nonsmokers. One particularly powerful carotenoid is lycopene. Lycopene is found in tomatoes and everything made from them including pizza sauce and ketchup. You will also find lycopene in watermelon guava and pink grapefruit.

Include them in your diet along with a little bit of fat as they are fat soluble. Most carotenoids are not damaged by cooking. The color is the most important key in identifying fruits and vegetables that will provide the most benefit. You might be surprised to know that red leaf lettuce has more carotenoids than iceberg lettuce just as there is more benefit from pink grapefruit than white.

The Last Weight-loss Program You Will Ever Need

Flavonoids are a serendipity because they are found in just about every plant from apples to onions and soy and even black and green tea contain flavonoids that help fight cancer.

Get the most benefit from flavonoids try these tips:

Sip wine. Drinking a little wine each day as well as tea. Have your cup of coffee first thing in the morning, then switch to tea for the remainder of the day. Combine fruits and make a fruit salad (fresh only). Buy a variety and vary different combinations. Add finely grated orange or lemon peel to fruit drinks, carbonated drinks and on salads, vegetable and even meats.

Tannins are not just colorful substances used in dying, making ink or tanning leather. Ellagic acid, one form of tannin, is in foods that stain. Strawberries, raspberries and blackberries. Get more tannins into your system and fight cancers, heart disease and stroke. Skip juices and go for the whole fruits. Check the labels of your jams and jellies and select according to which have a higher content of real fruit. This is more than likely the premium brands. Top off your food with a few berries to work them into your daily eating habits. Sprinkle them over cereal, pancakes and desserts.

Supplements – Is taking supplements beneficial? Visit your local supermarket, drugstore or health food store and you will find rows upon rows of vitamins and supplements. Each is minutely measured giving you the RDAs, DVs, IUs, milligrams and so on. It's enough information to make your head swim!

Some studies suggest that specific vitamin and mineral supplements can help reduce your risk of heart disease by 30 to 40 percent and even slow the progress of the disease according to Jeffrey Blumberg, M.D. associate director and chief of the Antioxidants Research Laboratory at the U.D. Department of Agriculture Human Nutrition Research Center on Aging in Boston. They are relatively inexpensive and easy to obtain over the counter.

Vitamins are also credited with boosting the immune system and it is believed that older people who take vitamin and mineral supplements do have stronger immune systems.

Generally speaking, the immune system begins to decline around age 50 and by age 60 may already be seriously compromised. The belief is that if your immune system can't protect you, the door is thrown wide open for cancer and other serious diseases to waltz right in.

So, the answer is yes, supplements can help but don't expect them to work miracles. You can't continue to do the steak and eggs or burger and fries thing and think that popping a pill will be a cure-all because it isn't!

If you are over 55, vitamin supplements will help prevent disease even though it may take at least six months to a year to register the improvement. That's not an excuse to put it off, because the sooner you begin, the better the results.

Let's take a look at weight for instance. If you take in too many calories and gain weight you increase the risk of cancer, heart disease and stroke. But, cutting the calories to either lose or maintain your weight may result in deficiencies in vitamins and minerals. You can replace key vitamins and minerals lost by dieting with carefully selected supplements.

Another challenge is compensating as the body's systems begin to slow down. As we age, our systems are not working as efficiently as they once were. For example, you don't have as much stomach acid that helps to get nutrients from food. That means that as much as 40% of the nutrients you ingest may go unused resulting in deficiencies of vitamins D, B6, B12, riboflavin, folate and calcium.

Your body's system for storing the nutrients isn't as efficient either because the percentage of body fat increases with age. While your metabolism keeps you alive and healthy, it also produces by products that can be harmful including free radicals and other compounds that cause damage to cells' DNA and can lead to many of the effects of old age.

As we get older, the body reduces the amount of antioxidants it produces and it will become more difficult to get enough antioxidant protection just from your food. Although you can get most of the nutrients you need from a multi-vitamin, you may want to take extra supplements of certain vitamins and minerals to promote optimum health.

As a cautionary measure, however, make certain that you are not exceeding the recommended ranges. You can get too much of a good thing. It is also advisable to consult with your physician regarding any supplemental regimen as some supplements may have adverse interaction with certain medications you are taking.

While we won't delve into the vast subject of supplements here, there are a few suggestions we would like to share with you.

Avoid multi-vitamins with time release formulas. By the time they dissolve they may be too far down the intestinal tract where absorption is poor.

Store your vitamins away from hot or humid places. It is better to keep them with your spices rather than the bathroom or near direct sunlight or heat.

Take your vitamins with a meal. Some nutrients are only released with fat so taking them with your low-fat meal is optimum.

Check the expiration date on the bottle. Buying a large amount just to save a few dollars isn't a bargain if you won't be using them before their effectiveness expires.

If you drink even moderately, take extra vitamins and minerals.

If you want to lose weight, take more calcium. If you don't consume enough calcium your body will over produce calcitriol. This hormone promotes fat storage in the body. But, calcium supplements won't be as beneficial as dietary calcium. Have four daily servings of nonfat or low-fat dairy products.

MANAGING YOUR ENVIRONMENT

Are you under the assumption that pollution is a modern day problem? Think again. In ancient times, the Greeks AND the Romans spewed huge amounts of toxins into the air extracting silver from lead.

The stench of an abandoned canal in Washington, D.C. clogged with animal carcasses and human waste was so bad it permeated the White House.

More than 70,000 chemical compounds were developed during the second half of the twentieth century. Many are credited with causing cancer in laboratory animals.

So, does this affect the risk of developing cancer, heart disease or stroke beyond age 60? You better believe it does and while there are varied opinions, there are researchers who believe that as much as 25% of all cancers could be prevented if Americans reduces exposure to smog, pesticides, second hand smoke and other hazards that we breathe, drink, eat and absorb into our bodies. While there are many factors that cause cancer, heart disease and stroke that we have no control over such as heredity, our environment is something we can do something about.

It's a killer – If you are a typical male smoker in your sixties or seventies, you began smoking at age 17 and have smoked about 27 cigarettes a day for 51 years. If you are a woman in the same range, you began smoking at around 24 and have been smoking 20 cigarettes a day for 45 years. And you have probably tried at least once or twice to quit like 80% of people who smoke.

Is it too late to quit? Absolutely not. Putting out that last cigarette as late as 60 to 80 can halt many of the worst effects of smoking. Yet 46% of older smokers don't believe that smoking is that harmful or that quitting at this stage in their life is worthwhile. If you fall into that category consider this:

- ☐ Within eight hours of quitting, your pulse rate and blood pressure drop and oxygen levels in your body will rise.
- ☐ Within 24 hours of quitting, your risk of a heart attack decreases.
- ☐ After one month, your circulation improves, your energy levels

surge and your lung function expands by up to 30%.

- [ ] After one year, your risk of heart disease is half that of someone who continues to smoke.

- [ ] After five years, your risk of having a stroke begins to decline .

- [ ] After 10 years, your chances of developing lung cancer are the same as that of someone who has never smoked.

Each time you take a puff you inhale more than 4,700 chemicals that have been shown to have effect throughout your body. Some of the milder effects are accelerated wrinkling of the skin, yellowing of the teeth and fingers and slower healing of wounds.

Here is a list of a few of those chemicals and what their common uses are:

Acetone	paint stripper
Ammonia	floor cleaner
Arsenic	ant poison
Butane	lighter fluid
Cadmium	car batteries
Carbon monoxide	car exhaust
Formaldehyde	morgue preservative
Methanol	anti-freeze
Naphthalene	mothballs
Nicotine	insecticide
Polonium 210	radioactive substance

The Last Weight-loss Program You Will Ever Need

Then along come the really dangerous effects of smoking including increasing the risk of disabilities like osteoporosis, hip fractures, cataracts, diabetes, tooth loss, and emphysema.

Smoking causes fatal complications. Every year, more than 400,000 Americans die of smoking related causes. That adds up to more than 1,000 a day making this the most preventable cause of death in the United States. 50% of those deaths are caused by cardiovascular disease and 30% by lung cancer.

Smoking hurts your heart. If you quit your risk of a heart attack is reduced by 50% in one year.

Smoking tops the list of cancer risks. If you quit even at age 65, your risk of developing lung cancer by age 75 is less than half of someone who continues to smoke.

Smoking is an addiction plain and simple. Don't blame yourself if you have tried several times to quit and failed. The prime ingredient in tobacco is Nicotine and is one of the most addictive drugs known to mankind. Is it hopeless? No. Many people have quit and so can you.

This is not a book about smoking cessation, but here are a few tips to help you.

Set a quit date and stick to it. Experts report that those who set a definite date are more likely to stick with it. Avoid stressful times like holidays and don't pick a date that is months away.

Quit cold turkey. If you do it this way, you will probably have a week to 10 days of withdrawal but then you'll be almost over the hump.

The Last Weight-loss Program You Will Ever Need

Throw them away. On the date you quit, throw away all tobacco products. Every hidden cigarette should be ferreted out and disposed of. Get rid of lighters, matches and ashtrays as well.

Banish alcohol. Alcohol can affect your resolve and make it easier to light up again. You don't have to quit alcohol forever, but spend at least of month of abstinence after you quit smoking.

Be prepared to fight the urges. As you go through withdrawal expect one or more of the following symptoms: upset stomach, difficulty concentrating, drowsiness, insomnia and irritability.

Once the nicotine is flushed from your body the withdrawal symptoms will gradually subside but they will probably never go away totally. That's because one is never enough. If you smoke one you'll smoke a dozen or more.

Change your rituals.

Short circuit stress.

Quit early in the week.

Stay in a smoke free world.

Give yourself daily pep talks.

Make a deal and reward yourself

Save those bucks.

Stall for time – delay lighting up.

Stay hydrated.

Cut down on caffeine.

Eat breakfast.

Although going cold turkey is the best bet, if you must do it gradually, the important thing is to QUIT!

Does it come from Grandma? – Genetics seems simple but is so complex that many scientists are still baffled by some aspects of the process. Genes are composed of millions of encoded nitrogen molecules that carry all of your reproductive blueprints. Every day 100 trillion cells depend on genes to tell them what they are supposed to be doing. The genetic code is a set of tutorials that tells the cells how to work properly. If one of those instructions is wrong, it changes how the cell functions. These erroneous instructions cause disease if they prevent the cell from doing the job it was designed to do and can cause the cell to die.

A genetic mistake is called a mutation. Having a mutation does not mean that you are pre-determined to get a disease. It just tells you that you should be more cautious about monitoring your overall health.

For instance only 5% of breast cancer is hereditary. But among women who have a history of breast cancer AND carry either the BRCA1 or BRCA2 (BRCA means breast cancer) gene the lifetime risk of breast cancer is about 80%. Women who have an inherited breast cancer gene may contract the disease 10 to 15 years earlier but it's also true that almost half won't get breast cancer until after age 60.

For most people the likelihood of developing inherited forms of cancer are about as likely as being struck by lightning and winning the lottery on the same day. But if your family does seem prone to a particular disease, it may be worth taking some precautions.

If you have a parent who died of a heart attack or a sibling who died of stroke at a young age that is something to share with your doctor as well as make some lifestyle changes like exercising, eating properly and not smoking.

Genetic testing is now available, but at a very high cost. Unless there is dramatic evidence that points to potentially serious genetic predispositions in your family tree, you're much better off taking normal precautions by living healthy.

Your environment and disease – We all carry a degree of toxins in our cells. Take DDT for example. The use was banned in 1972 after research indicated the suspicion it contributed to breast cancer. But, traces of DDT remains in the foods we eat and the water we drink for more than 50 years, we all have trace amounts in bodies.

Trace amounts probably will not cause you harm, however, 30 chemicals have been proven to cause cancer in humans while another 400 have been shown to cause cancer in laboratory animals and are suspected of causing human tumors.

Pollution increases the risk of heart attack.

Breast cancer rates appear to be higher in industrial areas.

Certain cancers are more common among farmers who use Pesticides.

Radon is linked to lung cancer.

The damage created by these hazards increase as we age. The body gradually loses the ability to rid itself of toxins that can damage your lungs, kidneys, liver and other major organs.

Here are some tips to lower your intake of air born pollutants:

Stick to side streets as you walk for exercise.

Avoid outdoor activities during rush hour.

Live in a smoke-free environment.

Clean your indoor air with a HEPA filter.

Pay attention to local outdoor pollution alerts.

Try some of these hints to avoid pesticide poisoning:

Eat plenty of vegetables and soy products each day.

Reduce your intake of beef, pork and chicken.

Wash and peel all fruits and vegetables carefully.

Keep your kitchen free of pesticides.

Exercise – We all know it. Exercise is good for you but, if you are over 60, breeze on by the advertising that touts 'buns of steel.' Recent research indicates that moderate exercise will give you as much protection from disease as the extensive exercise regimens touted by those much younger than you.

Experts now tell us to use a two-part exercise program that includes aerobic exercise like walking or bicycling to condition your heart plus strength training exercises such as calisthenics and low-intensity weight lifting to build muscle and cut fat. To begin you should only exercise two or three times a week but should work toward at least five times a week.

Easing into a routine like this gradually should be your goal. By age 60 almost everyone has some degree of osteoarthritis, osteoporosis, joint irritation or lack of flexibility. Exercising lightly will not aggravate these conditions, but will actually help them.

Exercise will also keep your heart young, drive down high blood pressure, build up good cholesterol, improve balance, enhance sex life, increase mental acuity, elevate mood, control diabetes, decrease cancer risk, strengthen bones, ease joint pain and much, much more.

Get started properly. Get a physical so you know that your body's systems can handle additional physical stress.

Warm up for at least 10 to 15 minutes using slow-walking, stretches or light calisthenics. As you get older you body need to ease into exercise gradually because your system is down about one third and takes longer to warm up and cool down.

Exercising more than 30 minutes at a time will help you lose weight if you do it three to five times a week and follow a proper diet. But if you don't need to lose weight, three 10 minute sessions each day will be beneficial for protection against disease.

Schedule a regular workout time. Dress for comfort. Have plenty of water along so as not to dehydrate.

Half of your exercise routine should include aerobics and the best aerobic exercise is walking, especially if you are over 60. Start out by timing yourself and gradually increasing the distance over time. Keep your pace constant, slow down on hills and track the temperature. If it's hot or humid your workout will seem harder. As you become more comfortable with your routine, try some variation like shortening steps, trying weights or swing your arms as you walk.

Here are some basic guidelines to follow for strengthening exercises:

Keep it slow – perform exercises slowly spending two seconds in the lifting phase of each exercise and four to six seconds in the lowering part. Moving too fast reduces the benefits and you could actually hurt yourself.

Always inhale before lifting, exhale while lifting and inhale as you lower the weight to get the best benefit.

Select just a few exercises to begin with, a few for the upper body and a few for the lower body. You can always increase as your routine helps you to gain stamina.

Use music to help establish a rhythm.

Pick the right kind of shoes. Walking or running shoes absorb the shock of your stride because of a slightly elevated heel that also helps prevent injuries to leg muscles and tendons. Tennis and other types of athletic shoes absorb impact of sideways movement and quick turns. Buy new shoes often even though they may last for years. That is because the shock absorption only lasts for a few months.

Wear loose fitting clothing for comfort, don't drink coffee or any diuretics before or while exercising and exercise vigorously enough so that you can't talk and exercise at the same time!

ATTITUDE AND AGING

Thankfully, researchers are finally beginning to understand and accept the link between mind and body. Even though the physiological make up of emotions themselves have not yet been identified, some researchers suspect that a small portion of the brain called the insular cortex may be the key.

The insular cortex regulates the autonomic nervous system which controls the automatic functions of our body such as breathing heartbeat and blood pressure. It also plays a role in higher brain functions and helps to process anger, fear, joy, happiness and sexual arousal.

Laboratory experiments with animals indicate that when the insular cortex is stimulated for long periods of time, causes a kind of damage to the heart muscle that is similar to sudden cardiac death. Other experiments with people who have epilepsy who were undergoing brain surgery that exposed the insular cortex found that stimulating the area with mild electrical pulses changed the person's heart rate and blood pressure.

Is it any wonder, therefore, that years of sorrow, anger and other negative emotions may cause a malfunction of the insular cortex? The research continues.

Whatever happens in that six inches between your ears, one thing is certain. Optimism, laughter, love and other positive emotions can counteract many harmful effects at any age, even in your sixties, seventies, eighties and beyond!

A happy outlook appears to trigger the release of endorphins. Endorphins relax the cardiovascular system and cytokines which alert the immune system to pay attention in detecting abnormalities like cancer cells.

The University of California, Riverside began a research project in 1921 whereby they followed the aging process of over 1,500 people who were preteens when the study began. The researchers concluded that among those subjects, such positive attributes as dependability, trust, agreeableness and open-mindedness were associated with a two to four year increase in life expectancy.

Let's explore some tips for developing a better outlook on your world.

Listen carefully to yourself. If you have put yourself down since childhood, over a lifetime negative subliminal message can take their toll by turning you into a pessimist. Spend one week writing down the phrases you use in your "self talk." Chances are you will find that you repeat a dozen or so phrases over and over again that reinforce that negative image. If you know about them, you can change them.

If an issue is not resolved it will continue to plague you and you will relive the negative emotions tied to that issue over and over again. Write yourself a letter spending about 20 minutes a day for four days and write about what you feel. Forget grammar, punctuation and so on. No one else will see this but you and you can throw it away when finished. Once you begin to write, don't stop until the time is up. This exercise will help you organize your thoughts and get them out of your system. By the end of the four days most people feel much better about themselves.

Seek out new challenges and opportunities. Always have something that is a goal just over the horizon. When you begin to close the gap and reach that goal, set another and another. Keep yourself consistently moving ahead.

Try and do one new thing every week or month. Visit a museum, go to the zoo, go to a book signing or lecture. The goal here is to eliminate monotony which is a sure killer of optimism.

Look for a new marvel of nature each day. Discover an abundance of happiness. Spoil your pet or if you don't have one, visit the human society and adopt one. Learn to laugh at yourself. Allow yourself to experience grief but don't let it control you.

Find someone who is worse off than you and lend a hand. Volunteer at a hospital, visit a nursery or a shelter.

In a preliminary study, researchers at the Institute of HeartMath in Boulder Creek, California, a biomedical research center that examines mind-body connections, asked 30 men and women to think for five minutes of either a compassionate moment in their lives or a time when they were upset or angry. "We found that simply recalling one episode of anger depresses the immune system for up to seven hours – but one episode of feeling compassion or caring enhances the immune system for about the same amount of time," says Jerry Kaiser, the Institute's director of health services.

Armed with that information, stop for a moment and think about how often you feel either end of that emotional spectrum. Makes you think a bit deeper about how we have the power to actually destroy ourselves through our emotions, doesn't it?

Here are a few quick tips for increasing joy, hope and optimism that will work no matter what your age:

Make a list of at least 50 great things that happen to you every day.

Laugh a lot. You'll heal your body and your mind.

Discover a new challenge each month.

Try meditating for just five minutes each day.

Sex After 50 – Ha! How many of you jumped ahead to this section? It's not surprising if you did and hopefully we can lend some positive reinforcement to certain cultural myths.

The importance of physical intimacy actually depends on the couple. An alarming number of men used to give up on sex after 60 and many women used to feel that their six life ended with menopause. Thankfully, that is no longer the case.

Sex at middle age can actually become better and more satisfying than ever before. Maturity gives a couple more experience in lovemaking. The children are usually grown and left home. The pressures of building a career and day to day life are usually less stressful than in younger years.

Our society places a disproportionate emphasis on youth, thus reinforcing the myth that older people have no sexual interest. People have a natural tendency to believe what society dictates and eventually just give up on sex after reaching middle age.

The Last Weight-loss Program You Will Ever Need

There are physiological changes that affect normal sexual function. Unfortunately people have taken these changes to mean that sexual function is over for them which needn't be the case at all.

Many men age 60 or over worry when they no longer have a spontaneous erection with visual stimulation. This doesn't mean that sexual function is over, but only means that they now require more direct stimulation. Sadly, many men will avoid intercourse until they have a spontaneous erection in fear that their wives will think they have a sexual problem.

As men get older they need longer periods of time between ejaculations and over 60 may require a full day or even several between ejaculations. This does not mean that he cannot enjoy intercourse and lovemaking in between.

Another serious problem exists where partners believe that climaxes are absolutely necessary. The male believes that he must have one and his female partner believes that if he does not he no longer finds her attractive.

Lack of lubrication is a problem for older women and impotence a problem for men. These are challenges that can be treated and should be discussed with your physician.

There are many factors that enter the equation when facing sexual problems. Medications, alcohol and major illness may be causing a lack of sexual desire. Again, all are potentially treatable and should be taken to your physician.

The most important tool any couple can put to use in their sexual relationship is the brain. Use it wisely and there is no reason why people over

50, 60, 70 and over should not have a healthy sexual relationship with their partner.

LAST MINUTE TIPS AND TRICKS

Some meat is good for you, but try and stick to these:

Eye of the round roast. A lean 3 ounce serving has 143 calories, 59 milligrams of cholesterol and just over 4 grams of fat. Protective nutrients include vitamins B12 and B6, zinc, niacin, potassium, riboflavin and magnesium.

Top loin steak. One lean 3 ounce serving with fat trimmed contains 168 calories, 65 milligrams of cholesterol and 7 grams of fat. Protective nutrients include vitamins B12 and B6, zinc, niacin, potassium, riboflavin and magnesium.

Lamb foreshank. One lean 3 ounce serving of the meat gives you 159 calories, 88 milligrams of cholesterol and 5 grams of fat. Protective nutrients include vitamin B12, zinc, niacin, riboflavin, magnesium and potassium.

Pork tenderloin. One lean 3 ounce serving contains 139 calories, 67 milligrams of cholesterol, and 4 grams of fat. Protective nutrients include vitamins B12 and B6, riboflavin, zinc and magnesium.

Supplement Smartly

Choose a high quality multivitamin.

Check the expiration date to make sure you will use it all in time.

Add an antioxidant supplement that contains 100 to 400 IU of vitamin E, 250 to 1,000 milligrams of vitamin C, 6 to 20 milligrams of beta-carotene, plus 70 to 100 micrograms of selenium.

Add a calcium supplement or be sure to get enough calcium through your diet. For women over age 50 and men over 65, take a total of 1,500 milligrams per day (1,000 milligrams a day for med aged 60 to 65). Be sure and take calcium in divided doses so that it is fully absorbed.

Buy a product that has equal percentages of the daily value for copper and zinc.

Choose a multivitamin that contains little or no iron.

Take your multivitamin and antioxidant supplements with meals or low-fat snacks to get the full benefit of fat and water soluble vitamins.

Buy dairy products that are fortified with vitamin D.

Do not take doses larger than those recommended by experts or without approval from your doctor.

Don't take calcium and your multivitamin supplement together.

Don't take calcium without checking with your doctor if you are on tetracycline.

Don't over consume magnesium products like certain laxatives, antacids and pain relievers if you have kidney problems.

Don't increase your consumption of supplements without checking with your doctor first, especially if you are on other medications.

Low Calorie Treats To Enjoy

3 Chocolate kisses – 75 calories, 4.5 grams of fat

24 fresh grapes – 81 calories, 0 grams of fat

1 cup fresh strawberries with 1 tablespoon powdered sugar – 86 calories, 0 grams of fat

½ cup of cranberry juice over ice with club soda and an organge slice - 91 calories, 0 grams of fat

5 vanilla wafers – 93 calories, 3 grams of fat

19 pieces of candy corn – 95 calories, 1.9 grams of fat

2 tablespoons low-fat yogurt topped with ½ cup of cherries and 2 teaspoons sliced almonds – 96 calories 3 grams of fat

2 cups air-popped popcorn tossed with 1 teaspoon melted margarine and 1 teaspoon honey - 97 calories, 3.8 grams of fat

½ cup sugar free instant pudding made with skim milk and ½ teaspoon shaved semi-sweet chocolate – 99 calories, 0.6 grams of fat

10 (1 inch) cubes of angel food cake topped with ¼ cup frozen raspberries in light syrup – 100 calories, 0 grams of fat

Health Screenings Are Important!

There are many health insurance programs that cover preventive health care like health screenings. Here are screenings that are important as you age:

Screenings for breast, cervical, vaginal, colorectal and prostate cancer including mammography.

Testing for loss of bone mass, which causes osteoporosis.

Diabetes monitoring and self-management.

Flu, pneumonia and Hepatitis B vaccinations.

Get your blood pressure checked annually.

Check your HDL and LDL cholesterol levels every year.

Get a Pap smear every year.

Use an inexpensive fecal occult-blood test to check for colon cancer.

Have a sigmoidoscopy done at least every three to five years or a colonoscopy done at least every 10 years.

Get a simple blood test to check for diabetes.

Check your skin often for changes to freckles and moles.

Don't just automatically get every test available to you. Discuss with your doctor the positive and negative aspects of certain tests.

Using Indoor Plants To Clean The Air

Lady palm, peace lily, ficus, golden pothos and areca palm are easy to grow, insect resistant and can absorb many of the cancer causing chemicals like benzene, arsenic and formaldehyde found in secondhand smoke and other household pollutants.

A normal houseplant can filter about six cubic feet of air or about the size of a overstuff chair. Position the plant on a table or floor beside your bed or favorite chair to maximize the amount of clean air in your breathing zone.

Don't Get Burned!

People over 65 account for half of all new cases of skin cancer. Damage to the skin doesn't happen overnight but accumulates over years.

Use a sunscreen with an SPF of at least 15.

Look for the UV Index in your local newspaper.

Wear a broad-brimmed hat and sunglasses in the sun.

Conduct a self-exam of your skin once a month looking for any new growths or changes in moles, freckles or birthmarks.

Don't be fooled by clouds. Sunlight and UV rays penetrate the clouds so wear sunscreen even on cloudy days.

Don't forget to apply sunscreen to ears, neck and the back of your hands.

****

BOOK THREE: MANAGING YOUR STRESS!

****

HOW TO REDUCE STRESS AT WORK & AT HOME

TABLE OF CONTENTS

INTRODUCTION

WHAT IS STRESS?

HOW TO CONTROL STRESS

SELF HYPNOSIS

OTHER STRESS REDUCERS

TAKE A STRESS TEST

CONFIDENCE AND SELF ESTEEM

FINAL THOUGHTS

THE LITTLE TEST

INTRODUCTION

Did you know that 90% of doctor visits are for stress related symptoms?

Stress bombards us every day from all directions. Maybe it's sitting in the midst of highway gridlock when you are already late for an important appointment. Or how about the bill you forgot to pay? It could be a phone call from the school complaining about your child's behavior.

These are just the annoying little stress triggers that we handle every day. What about the larger issues? Retirement, moving, divorce or, heaven forbid, the death of a loved one or friend can come out of the blue and here comes the stress launching you into treading murky waters one more time.

The impression is that the feelings of stress come from outside sources when, in reality, it happens inside of us.

When we feel as though we are under pressure, our bodies react the same way that we have trained them to do with a rise in blood pressure, tightening of muscles and accelerated breathing.

These physical symptoms are generally referred to as "fight or flight" responses. This is a term leftover from historical times when the choices were to flee or stand and fight.

Unfortunately, today we don't have those options. Each situation must be dealt with and that's where the stress comes in. Some stress is unavoidable and is actually good for you as we will discuss further on. But too much stress leads to troubles that can range from upset stomach to anxiety attacks and even as serious as heart attacks.

There's a whole arsenal of stress busting tools available that we will discuss here. Hopefully, the more you understand your stress, the better prepared you are at controlling your body's response to stress and restoration to a calmer state of mind.

WHAT IS STRESS?

Chemically, stress is a condition that your body enters as the result of a message received from your brain telling it to prepare to run or fight. The body reacts by preparing for that eventuality. The brain tells the adrenal glands to send a rush of two hormones (adrenaline and noradrenaline) to the muscles in preparation for them to respond to a fear or a threat.

It is the job of the brain to protect the body. It accomplishes this by telling the noradrenaline to redirect blood flow from lower priority areas of your body (like skin or your abdomen) to the muscles to give you a "power boost."

At the same time the brain is also telling the adrenaline to speed up your breathing to take in more oxygen to feed the work being done on the muscles with the noradrenaline.

Unfortunately, when you can't make a decision about how to react (fight or flight), these two hormones are caught in limbo rushing around madly waiting for you to decide what you want them to do. Since you aren't doing that, the only choice they have is to cause vomiting, make you tremble, panic or maybe even pass out.

It's actually a very efficient process and has worked wonderfully for thousands of years. When we were running across the plains barefoot with a spear in our hand bearing down on supper, we needed this process to protect us. Indeed, the entire system is just the result of the brain doing what it is supposed to do. . .keep the body functioning and protect it.

We no longer chase the wooly mammoth nor does our survival revolve around running away from a rival tribe (well maybe just a little). The battles today are demanding employers, uncontrollable traffic, annoying neighbors, partners, children and oh yes, taxes!

Here's where the interesting part of this analysis comes in. Even though our situation has changed, the chemicals are still there along with the vehicle to drive them.

The system is very efficient and works quite effectively. This is why you have stress. It is merely a response to a perceived threat and the brain will set it in motion on a subconscious level even at the slightest sensation of danger. In fact it will DEMAND this action.

Since we now live in an "enlightened" society, we are conditioned not to throw a spear at the boss, strangle your spouse or set the neighbor's house afire.

What is needed is the ability to change our programmed responses. We need to discern the difference between real threats and our own internalized perceptions of danger. Sounds pretty simple, huh?

Sure it does. Until you're sitting in that freeway gridlock, half an hour late for the most important career busting appointment of your life, knowing full well that your blankety blank boss will turn the account over to that jerk in the office and you'll never get the raise you were counting on when your son starts college in the fall. . . .whew!

Here come the chemical twins, adrenaline and noradrenaline ready to do battle with no battle to go to. They're rushing through your body and have got to attack something. Your muscles aren't responding by running or fighting so they'll just pick any old organ to attack instead. A good one is the heart.

Sometimes a dose of the chemical twins is a good thing. After all, even though we are now "civilized" there are still very real threats in the world. Just take a look at the evening news or read about the latest "mugging" in the newspaper.

So, here is the paradox. You need the chemical twins to protect you from real danger but you don't need them to cause illness, unhappiness and stress. The challenge is knowing when to have them and you don't need them.

Logically you know that you don't need them under most normal situations like: at work, at a party or when the kids are screaming in your ear.

So what can you do? Some people turn to drugs or alcohol and others take out their frustration on the people they care about the most. You can learn how to control the twins. Let's do that now.

HOW TO CONTROL STRESS

What's causing your stress?

A slow buildup of everyday annoyances: a dead car battery, traffic jam, buttons that pop off your clothes as you are going to an important meeting. It's the little things that get under your skin

Is it a tight schedule and seemingly insurmountable problems? Bills to pay, a boss to please, a colicky baby to pacify? Juggling many roles is a main cause of stress.

Maybe it's positive and negative life changes, from the joy of a wedding to the loss of a spouse; from the exhilaration of a job promotion to sadness at moving away from old friends.

Perhaps the cause of your stress is inner conflict. Anger with your boss actually may be old anger against a parent bubbling to the surface. If you can recognize a pattern from the past, this can be an instant stress reliever. Take some time, even just 30 seconds and write down your feelings.

The Last Weight-loss Program You Will Ever Need

What you need to do is *relax*. Huh? It can't be that simple! Yes, it can and you can do it. No, we can't control other people and situations. What you can do is control how you respond to people and events.

What you have done is given away control to others. What you need to do is regain that control seal it up and only let the twins out when it's really necessary.

When was the last time you actually relaxed? Can you remember what it was like? Were you calm and collected? Was your breathing normal? Were your muscles loose? And, did you feel that way without any outside stimulants like drugs? If so, the good news is that you can restore that same feeling at will. Yes, you can definitely take it back whenever or wherever you choose.

When your mind is bypassing the chemical twins and sending truly relaxing messages to your body, wonderful things begin to happen. Just as the chemical twins jump to attention when you stress, other chemicals go to work when you relax causing you to have a feeling of contentment.

While relaxing, actions taken by people and external events are still important but not necessarily personal. You are able to discern that no one is launching a direct attack upon you or anyone or anything of yours.

Small problems remain small problems and not the wooly mammoth charging down upon you. Large events will become smaller and not cause you to get out of your car during gridlock and shout obscenities to the drivers in front of you.

Those people who are horrible and annoying, shrink to a caricature serving up no more significance in your world than an ant on a picnic table. As you continue your journey toward relaxation, you can watch these people with amusement. When you reach the point of total relaxation you are able to see your world as it is, not for how you feel about it.

Everything you do is a matter of choice. You choose to be angry, happy or indifferent. You make a conscious choice to take action or not to take action.

On the opposite end of the spectrum are the chemical twins controlling what you know is stress and you are bumped, pushed and thrown into chaos. No choice and no idea why you don't have a choice.

Obviously, relaxing is a good thing because it gives you choice. It puts you back in the drivers seat instead of the chemical twins.

So relax already! Sure, just like that.

Do you remember tormenting your neighbors cat as a child? You had the upper hand until kitty fought back. You'd step away from the torment and probably forget all about it until the next time you scratched. It took a few lessons, but pretty soon you understood if you tormented the cat, the cat would fight back. That was a conscious action taken to prevent being hurt. It was a survival strategy just like fight or flight, except that this was **behavior modification** instead of an automatic response.

As you grew older the behavior for survival changed but the bottom line is that you probably used a dozen behaviors without even thinking about it every day of the week. The one behavior that you probably overlooked is the most important one of all, the behavior to relax.

If relaxation is just another behavior that means it's a learned response. And, if that is the case you be able to change the behavior. Chances are you were never taught how to do that which is why you are reading this in the first place.

You have to teach your brain how to do it. Actually, your brain already knows how subconsciously, but you need to teach it how to do it consciously. In order to do that, you need an understanding of how your mind works.

Everything you have ever encountered or done in your entire lifetime is permanently recorded in your subconscious mind. Most of it is not remembered consciously. If I ask you, "How much is two and two," you will immediately answer, "four." That was from your conscious memory. But if I ask you what you had for dinner ten years ago tonight, it will more than like be impossible for you to consciously remember it at all. However, your subconscious remembers it in great detail.

When you drive your care, you are probably thinking about all kinds of things other than driving the car. Your subconscious, through habit, was controlling all your driving actions. You just automatically arrive at your destination without giving it detailed conscious thought.

You didn't have to think "push the brake" or "ease up on the gas pedal." You did it all automatically controlled by your subconscious. Your subconscious is designed to protect you. It controls all body functions. If you are cold in the night, it awakens you. If you need to go to the bathroom, it awakens you also. If you burn your hand, it will raise a blister to protect you. It controls your heartbeat and all other involuntary functions of the body.

Your subconscious doesn't rationalize, it doesn't ask questions, doesn't know truth from falsehood. It merely acts upon whatever information is stored within.

There are actually four states of consciousness, but for our purposes we will be dealing with just two:

Beta – this is our waking state

Alpha – first step to the subconscious

The Alpha state is where we will begin our work. This is the state where you are relaxed, the normal machinations of your conscious mind are just a little distant and you feel warm and comfortable. The chemical twins are sealed up where they belong

Have you ever sat in a car waiting for a friend or family member to run in and make a quick purchase or run an errand? It may be a warm, sunny, spring day. The window is open and you can feel a gentle breeze caress your cheek and fluff your hair. The sun feels warm and cozy on your face. Before you know it, your eyelids begin to droop as you sit and enjoy a moment of oneness with your surroundings. Not awake and not asleep you are totally relaxed and content to drift along quietly enjoying the sensation of the warm sun and the gentle breeze.

If you have ever had this or a similar experience, you were in that Alpha state. Close your eyes and see if you can recapture the same sensations you had while you were in that state. Take a few moments to do that then imagine a car door slamming and pulling your instantaneously back in to the Beta state. Wow! What a rude awakening.

This level is where you can do the best work for yourself on a subconscious level. This is also a state of meditation, and the level you work with using self-hypnosis.

The truth is that you are actually in this state every single day at least two times. Those times are the fleeting moments just before you drift off to sleep and just as you awaken.

Your conscious mind has the ability to reason out a course of action that would be helpful to you. However, the conscious mind needs the cooperation of the subconscious and will send its energy out to implement the decision.

Your energy source is the subconscious mind. No matter what you consciously do to instruct the subconscious mind to do something thee is no way to permanently override what the subconscious mind has been programmed to do.

Let's take a look at some examples. If a very young child is told by a parent, teacher, elder sibling or anyone else in a position of authority:

"You never do anything right."

"What's the matter with you?"

"Why can't you be more like Billy?"

"Don't you have a brain in your head."

"Why are you so stupid?"

"You will never amount to anything!"

This child will often be a failure in life. The reason is that this child's conscious mind is not developed enough to block this type of information. Therefore, it becomes a fact in his subconscious mind.

As he/she grow to adulthood, his subconscious will be a very good student and apply everything it has learned. Remember, the subconscious is not right or wrong, good or bad, it is merely a computer just like the one you are reading from now.

His subconscious will force the conscious to act in exactly the same manner that was programmed as a child.

The subconscious mind will only accept what the conscious mind believes at the time the suggestion is offered. However, if the conscious mind changes an opinion on a given matter after it has become embedded in the subconscious the subconscious will not change with it.

These factors are important to understand before you begin your work. There are certain "tapes" in your subconscious mind that will not be changed. What you can do is create "new" responses.

SELF HYPNOSIS

Now that you have a very basic understanding of how the conscious and subconscious mind work, your first step is to learn how to put your mind in this state yourself in order to facilitate the changes that need to be made. Since self-hypnosis is simple to learn we will begin with that modality and give you several examples that you can use for self-hypnosis.

The first thing you need to do is learn how to hypnotize yourself. There are three tools that you will be using: suggestion, concentration and imagination. If you have a good imagination you will have no trouble mastering these techniques very quickly.

It is important not to try too hard. The whole concept is to just relax and let yourself go. If you try too hard you will become tense and this is exactly what you don't want.

Also ignore any analytical attitude. If you don't, you will keep the conscious mind awake and the whole object of hypnotizing yourself is to relax.

We assume you want to hypnotize yourself or wouldn't be doing this. You can't go into self-hypnosis against your will. Therefore you can't do it unless you follow the rules.

Before we begin, it is important to realize that there is no set "script" to the verbiage of a hypnotic trance. There are different techniques used by pioneers in hypnotherapy. The first technique was developed by one of those pioneers. His name was Charles Tebbetts who was already a teenager by World War I. Charles is known for his comment that, "all hypnosis is self-hypnosis, and the power is in the mind of the person being hypnotized."

Our first technique is called "Fractional Relaxation," and is one of the best induction methods for beginners. It takes a little longer than some other formulas, but it's a great conditioning technique for faster methods which can be more easily learned later. It relaxes the body completely, often to the point of partial or total loss of bodily awareness. Tension is released and the conscious mind drifts I and out of awareness of the surroundings, often viewing mental images of forgotten events from the subconscious.   Here's how you do it:

BEGIN INDUCTION

Lie down on your back, arms parallel to your body, fingers loosely outstretched and palms downward. Separate the feet by eight or ten inches so that no part of your thighs are touching. Use a pillow if you wish, and make yourself as comfortable as possible. Remove or loosen clothing that binds you in any way and remove your shoes if they are tight. The idea is to get comfortable and relaxed.

If you are recording this procedure, use the second person throughout, but if you intend to use it without a recording, memorize it in the first person. It is given here in the second person so it may be read directly fro the book into the microphone. Start reading in a soft voice, rather slowly, and gradually slow down more and more, drawing out your words and pausing often between sentences. Your voice and the pace of your speech must suggest drowsiness and relaxation. Speak in a very slow monotone.

Now let's assume you are in the described position, and are listening to your voice coming from your recorder. He is what you should hear:

"Fix your eyes on a spot on the ceiling and take three long, deep breaths. Inhale, hold the air in your lungs for three seconds, and as you exhale slowly, you will relax all over. Now let's take the first breath. Inhale. (pause) Exhale – Sleep now (pause) Now another deep breath, even deeper than before. Inhale. (pause) Exhale – Sleep now. (pause) Now another deep breath, even deeper than before. Inhale. (pause) Exhale – Sleep now. (pause) Now as your whole body begins to relax, and as every muscle and nerve begins to grow loose and limp – your eyelids also become heavy and tired. They grow heavier and heavier, and will close now. The lids have become so tired and so heavy, it would be difficult to open them, but have no desire to try because you want them to remain closed until I tell you to open them. (pause)

Now I want you to concentrate all of your attention on your right foot. Relax the toes of your right foot. Imagine they are like loose rubber bands dangling from your foot. (pause) Let this loose feeling spread back through the ball of the foot, and then all the way back to the heel. (pause) (Drag out the word all and speak very slowly fro this point on, pausing between ALL sentences.)

Now let this relaxed feeling go up into the calf of the leg. Let the calf muscles go loose-and-limp and LA-A-A-ZY. (long pause) And now, while your muscles and nerves are relaxing, let your mind relax also. Let it drift away to pleasant scenes in your imagination. Let your mind wander where it will, as you go deeper – deeper into drowsy relaxation. You are breathing easily; all of your cares and tensions are fading away, as you go deeper – d-e-e-p-e-r into drowsy slumber. Every breath that you take – every noise that you hear makes you go deeper, deeper, into pleasant, comfortable relaxation.

Now let the wonderful wave of relaxation move from your right calf up into the large thigh muscles. Let them go loose and limp. The right leg is now completely relaxed and comfortable. (pause) Now the left foot. The toes relax, the whole foot relaxes just as the right one did – limp and lazy. Let the feeling of pleasant relaxation go up into the left calf. Let the calf muscles go. Your legs are feeling heavy like pieces of wood. As you relax the left thigh muscles, they feel heavier and heavier and you become more and more drowsy. Now as the wave of relaxation moves upward through your hips and abdomen, you let go more and more. Think of your abdomen as an inflated ball. Your are letting the air out of the ball and it spreads out and relaxes completely. Stomach and solar plexus relax. Let them go – as you go further into deep – deep slumber. (pause)

(slowly) The fingers in your right hand are now relaxing and so is your wrist. Now your forearm relaxes. On up to your right shoulder – your whole right arm is relaxed and numb. You probably feel your fingers or your toes tingling. This is a good sign, so continue to go deeper. And now, just go on over, into a deep, deep hypnotic sleep. (pause)

The fingers on your left hand are completely relaxed. Your hand and forearm are letting go. Up, through your elbow, to your upper arm, relax. Now the left shoulder, let go – loose, limp and lazy. Now relax all the large back muscles, from your shoulders all the way down to your waist – let them all go limp and loose. (Remember, plenty of pauses. Continue to speak softly and very slowly.)

Relax the muscles in your neck. Let your jaws separate and let the chin and cheek muscles go loose and rubbery. (pause) Now let your eyes go. Let them go completely – relax and feel comfortable and good. Relax the eyebrows too and the forehead. Let the muscles rest. Back across the scalp – let the entire scalp relax – from the forehead all the way back to the back of the neck –

all relaxed – all resting – all loose. You are now completely relaxed. Your body feels boneless. You are going deeper and deeper into restful hypnosis. Your mind is experiencing a wonderful feeling of tranquility. Your subconscious is now receptive to the helpful suggestions I am now going to give it. (At this point the suggestion is given to the subconscious mind.)"

END INDUCTION

What we are using in this next example is a variation of the Fractional Relaxation Technique called the "Rapid Induction Technique."

BEGIN INDUCTION

1.   Make yourself as comfortable as you can on a mat, a couch or a chair.

2.   Inhale deeply and exhale, releasing all muscular tensions everywhere in the body. Continue to breathe naturally, easily and gently.

3.   Close your eyes. Focus your attention gently on your subconscious mind and give it the following commands silently and in sequence:

a.   Address yourself by name. (The name or nickname to which you usually respond to automatically when called by another person. Say silently to your subconscious mind, "I WANT YOU TO RELAX, VERY DEEPLY, NOW!"

b.   Let go and let down. Feel your mind, your emotions and your physical body sink quickly and deeply into relaxation, drifting ever deeper and deeper until you reach a plateau of relaxation.

c.   At this point, again address your subconscious mind by name and once more say silently to yourself, "I WANT YOU TO RELAX MORE DEEPELY, NOW!"

    d.   Feel yourself plunging deeper into relaxation, going down further and deeper until you reach another plateau of relaxation.

    e.   Once again, address your subconscious mind quietly, silently, by name and repeat the command, "I WANT YOU TO RELAX MORE DEEPLY NOW!"

    f.   And finally, once more, address yourself in a silent whisper, calling yourself by name and giving yourself a final command, "I WANT YOU TO RELAX MORE DEEPLY NOW!"

    g.   At this time you should reach a very effective level of deep relaxation when you can give yourself very effective suggestions toward achieving your desired goals.

    h.   You may give yourself suggestions in the form of visualizations, positive verbal suggestions, altered feelings or emotions such as:

        1) Visualizing your ideal configuration and weight.

        2) Replacing any fears, anxieties, depressions or other negative feelings by a sense of self confidence, optimism, pride or other positive emotion through verbal suggestions and suggested feelings.

        3) Permitting a feeling of deep pervasive peace to envelop you.

        4) Suggesting to your subconscious mind – time contractions

– for example, that the next hour will seem like only ten minutes have passed.

5) Any other suggestions consistent with your selected goals.

4. With daily practice for about two weeks, using this Rapid Self Induction Technique, you should be able to put yourself into an effective level of deep relaxation, within 30 seconds whether lying down, sitting or standing up.

5. After you have mastered the Rapid Self Induction Technique, with an additional 1 to 3 weeks of daily practice to achieve a state of deep, effective relaxation within 1 to 5 seconds merely by closing your eyes and silently saying to yourself, "RELAX." This almost instant self induction should be practiced consistently in all positions (lying, sitting and standing) to maintain proficiency.

END INDUCTION

Now that you have learned how to induce an advanced state of relaxation, you must learn how to structure the suggestion you would like to teach to your subconscious mind.

The subconscious mind must obey suggestions as though they were orders. While in hypnosis, with the conscious mind somewhat inhibited, it is possible to reach the subconscious mind directly with the suggestions that you want it to program.

It is very important to understand that the subconscious operates without the benefit of your conscious reasoning. Therefore you must be extremely careful with wording your suggestions. Structure them correctly and the subconscious will carry them out for you faithfully without conscious effort of any sort. Your motivation must be strong.

Start your suggestion with your motivating desire:

"Because I have a strong desire to live stress free, highway gridlock no longer upsets me"

"Because I have a strong desire to have an attractive, slim figure and because I enjoy wearing a size nine dress my body no longer requires more calories than it needs to live healthy"

There are examples of two complete auto suggestions. A couple of factors are important. You must always phrase the suggestion in the present tense as if the action has already occurred. You must never mention the negative behavior you wish to eliminate.

Suggest action not the ability to act. In other words, don't say, I have the ability to live stress free. . . .and so on. You must be specific.

Use repetition when writing your suggestion. Repeat it, enlarge upon it and repeat it again in different words. Embellish it with convincing adjectives. Repeat your suggestion daily until it becomes entrenched in your subconscious.

OTHER STRESS REDUCERS

Research has shown that the stress hormone cortisol reduces a person's ability to retrieve information and memory. Even worse, this same stress hormone is linked to progressive shrinking of the hippocampus – an important memory center in the temporal region. High levels of stress also promote depression, which severely impairs memory and increases the risk for dementia.

To reduce stress, try relaxation exercises. Sit quietly and breathe deeply and slowly. Relax each part of your body, starting with the top of your head and finishing with your toes. Look for humor in tense situations and talk about your feelings with family members, friends or a therapist, if necessary.

Try reducing stress and anxiety with fresh, natural scents. In general they induce a calming state. In one recent study, volunteers became extremely anxious when they were confined in coffin-like tubes, but then calmed down when the tubes were infused with the smells of green apple and cucumber. These odors seem to have an impact on the limbic systems, the emotional center of the brain.

If you anticipate a situation where you will feel anxious, wash your hair that morning with a green-apple-scented shampoo and/or dab a bit of the shampoo in a cloth to take with you.

Here are a few tips that will lower stress in five minutes or less:

- Move around.
- Take a quick trip through the halls of your workplace, or
- Walk around the block.
- Walk up and down a flight of stairs.
- Do 15 jumping jacks
- Stretch while seated at your desk. Lace your fingers under your knee

and draw it to your chest. Repeat with the other knee. This stretches the leg and lower back.

☐ Next, stretch your arms above your head, palms up and fingers interlaced. Drop your hands to your sides, then raise your right shoulder to your right ear, keeping your head vertical. Repeat this stretch with the left shoulder. Finally, bend back the fingers of each hand. This is especially important if you use a computer for long periods.

☐ Take 10 long deep breaths. Your belly should expand as you inhale and contract as you exhale.

☐ Massage your eyes and ears. Place your palms over your eyes. Slowly spiral your palms while applying gentle pressure. Do the same for your ears. Blocking out all sights and sounds, even for just a few seconds, is a psychologically refreshing experience.

☐ Try aromatherapy. Put a drop of lemon-lime or orange essential oil in a saucer. These gently scents relax you without making your home or office smell like an incense store.

☐ Get the best sleep. Early morning sleep is really the most restful sleep you can get. Men sent to bed at 2:15 a.m. and awakened at 6:15 a.m. slept more soundly than ones sent to bed at 10:30 and awakened at 2:30 a.m. So, if you are stressed and can get only four hours of sleep, stay up as late as possible to get the most benefit from your limited sleep. This does not replace a full night's sleep. Resume normal sleep pattern as quickly as possible.

Meditation is a favorite stress buster for some people. Taking time every day to disengage from the demands of the world can ease your mind and your body into a deeply relaxed state – the opposite of the stress response.

Meditation fosters your ability to step back from life and observe the passing scenery and your own thoughts in a detached manner. Studies have linked the regular practice of meditation to reductions in anxiety, work-related stress. . .and blood pressure, too.

There are many meditation techniques, but here is one that is simple:

- ☐ Sit quietly and comfortably in a place where you will not be disturbed.

- ☐ Focus your attention on your breathing.

- ☐ Feel the breath as it comes into your nose. . .and when it goes out.

- ☐ Other thoughts will enter your mind. Just observe them and let them go. Return your attention to your breath.

Start practicing meditation for five to 10 minutes a day, gradually increasing it to 20 to 30 minutes. Keep a clock nearby so you can keep track of the time. Caution! A clock alarm or kitchen timer is too jarring. Some people, however, set their wristwatch alarms.

Physical activity neutralizes the fight-or-flight response, easing tension and anxiety and leaving you invigorated. Regular moderate exercise reverses much of the damage caused by stress and can also improve immune system function, lower blood pressure and improve your mood.

Intense aerobic exercise – running or aerobics classes at a gym – is an effective stress buster, but so is more relaxed walking.

Do what you want to do – any exercise that you find enjoyable – and do it for at least 20 minutes every day. More, however, is not always better.

Human beings have an inborn affinity for nature. There is a scientific name for it "biophilia." Contact with scenes of nature and living things has been shown to reverse the effects of stress. For example:

- ☐ Employees whose windows look out on trees and grass report less work stress than those with views of parking lots.
- ☐ An aquarium in a dentist's waiting room lowers anxiety.
- ☐ Eating lunch on a park bench will relax your body.
- ☐ Spending a half hour in your garden will make your work worries recede into the distance.
- ☐ If you live in a city, consider a back to nature vacation a week in the mountains will recharge your batteries more deeply than a short stroll in the park.
- ☐ Let a little piece of nature into your daily life – get a pet. Persian cat, parakeet or beagle. It doesn't really matter what type of pet. Pet owners are healthier and respond better to stress than other folks.

Reduce stress and tension with humor. Being able to take yourself and your life less seriously is the stress antidote par excellence. How tense can you be when you're laughing at yourself?

Try looking for the lighter side of every situation. Indulge your taste for entertaining books and moves.

Does a newspaper cartoon tickle your funny bone? Tape it to your bathroom mirror as a reminder to lighten up.

The next time your spouse acts up, ask yourself, What would Groucho Marx have to say about this?

Have funny props around. Keep a clown nose in your glove compartment to transform a traffic jam into circus time. Why should kids have all the fun?

Cultivate your friendships. Close ties to others make you feel warm inside. . .and they also temper your body's reaction to stress. The world feels safer when you know that other people are on your side. Expressing your worries and troubles to a sympathetic ear often makes them easier to bear.

The mere presence of a friend blunts the pulse and blood pressure rise that accompany stressful tasks. People with many friends have lower cholesterol and stronger immune systems. They live longer than loners, too.

For short term periods of stress, follow a high carbohydrate, low protein diet. The carbohydrates deliver energy to the body. For longer stressful periods reverse the diet – that is, consume more protein and few carbohydrates. Other foods that fight stress are foods that are rich in vitamins C and A like raw carrots peppers and broccoli. There's a bonus as well, chewing crunchy foods helps to dissipate the tension.

How about some natural therapies for stress? Here are a few:

 ☐ **Lavendar -** Use the flowers. This is a beautiful herb and is widely used. Many do not realize that it is an effective treatment for headaches related to stress. Also good for depression.

- □ **St. Johns Wort** - Taken internally, has a sedative and pain reducing effect. Use in treatment of neuralgia, anxiety, tension and similar problems.

- □ **Vervain** - Also known as Wild Hyssop. Will strengthen the nervous system while easing depression and melancholia. Good for fever and best for colds, and for menopausal irritations.

Here are more tips to consider for reducing stress:

- □ This one is a "no-brainer" and we won't go into detail here, but if you are a smoker – STOP!

- □ Try to avoid tight deadlines, keep your schedule looser.

- □ Ask for help instead of insisting on doing it all yourself.

TAKE A STRESS TEST

The standard tests that doctors use to tell whether you are an easily stressed "hot reactor" (and at greater risk for disease) are pretty simple, so take your pick, says Frank Barry, M.D., a family practice physician in Colorado Springs and author of Make the Change for a Healthy Heart. For the first two tests, you'll want to take a blood-pressure reading twice – once before the test and once during the test – for comparison.

Test 1: Chill out. In Test 1, put your and into a bucket of cold water for one minute and have someone measure your blood pressure right after you have done it. If it goes up into the high range in response to physical stress, you are a "hot reactor."

Test 2: Do some math. Test 2 is a little more cerebral. Start with the number 100 and mentally subtract 7, then continue to subtract 7 until you get to 2. In the midst of your figuring, have your blood pressure taken. "There's no exercise, no threat to your life, but a lot of people still feel mental stress and their blood pressures soot up," says Dr. Barry.

Test 3: Talk to yourself. You can also test yourself without the shock of cold water or the mental anguish of math. As yourself: Are you working toward your own true goals or someone else's? If you are busy trying to keep up with the Joneses, "you're still in the rat race, even if you have retired. You're much more likely to feel the effects of stress regardless of whether you're a "hot reactor," says Dr. Barry.

CONFIDENCE AND SELF ESTEEM

The greatest challenges to your confidence come when you're facing a situation that *looks* impossible. When this happens, you must tap in to the unseen force of self-assurance so that you can press beyond supposed limits. It's not a matter of what things look like on the outside—the key is to recognize what you have working on the *inside*.

Confidence is often the missing link to seeing yourself accomplish the impossible. You just have to believe that you have what it takes to be successful, and don't back down from your capable stance.

The Last Weight-loss Program You Will Ever Need

You are in control of your thoughts. If you choose to believe you have confidence - that you're energized - then you will be. The next time you face a big challenge, take a deep breath and fill your heart with the belief that you have unlimited energy running through your veins. Build your confidence by reflecting on those things you've already accomplished. If you did it once, you can certainly do it again.

Today, receive the confidence you deserve—and you'll find that you always had it within you.

Don't confuse self-esteem with arrogance: Arrogance is an over evaluation of your worth, while self-esteem is a healthy opinion of yourself—it's valuing yourself to the point that you don't allow other people or negative situations and circumstance to influence the way you feel about yourself. Until you value yourself, you won't value anything, and other people won't value you either. After all, your relationship with yourself is the most important one you'll ever have.

When you're filled with self-doubt, give yourself a little pep talk. Repeat

"[Your name], you are great! You are a unique individual, a new kind of person the world has never known. You were born to do well. You were born to succeed. You were born to bless the lives of others. You were born to be great, and you have what it takes to be great. You are enthusiastic, optimistic, and a change-embracer. You are a giver, rather than a taker. You are organized. You are a hard worker. You are happy. You are a master over yourself, you are a leader. You are a big thinker. As blessed as you are with all these talents, there isn't one thing in the world you can't do. You will never fail. [Your name], go out and make today an 'attitude is everything' day!"

By making this profession every day, you'll experience an awesome self-esteem boost! Remember, you are priceless—your past is history, and your future is now!

FINAL THOUGHTS

Let's review some of what you have learned about stress. Steel will snap from it and a pressure cooker will blow its lid. Stress, pressure, tension is a fact of everyday life for most of us.

Remember that it puts you at risk for heart attack, stroke, insomnia, backache, headache, irritable bowel syndrome, sports injuries and infertility.

Stress can trigger serious illness like Graves disease and fibromyalgia. Stress even makes us more susceptible to the common cold.

With your health at stake, using some of the methods we have discussed is essential. Also, it's important that you remember that stress is a physiological response. It isn't all in your head! You owe it to yourself to take the time to use the stress-reducing techniques on a daily basis.

We've already given you a great selection, but we want to make certain that you have a wide range of coping skills to use at home, work and other places. So here are an additional 12 keys to stress reduction to help you open the door to a more relaxing life. They contain dozens of additional helpful hints. Choose those best suited for you.

Breathe deeply. Relax your muscles, expanding your stomach and chest. Exhale slowly. Repeat several times.

Follow your breath as it flows in and out. Do not try to control it. This is a good way to relax in the midst of any activity. This technique allows you to find a breathing pattern that is natural and relaxing to you.

Use this yoga technique: Inhale slowly, counting to eight. Exhale through your mouth, even more slowly, counting to sixteen. Make a sighing sound as you exhale, and feel tension dissolve. Repeat 10 times.

Exercise regularly. Aerobic exercise, such as walking and swimming, produces brain chemicals that uplift your mood and mental well-being. Exercise also improves sleep and gives you time to think and focus on other things. Beware of compulsive exercise, however.

Yoga is an age-old system for stretching and strengthening the muscles. Take a class or learn at home with a good book or video.

Neck and shoulder exercises are useful for the desk-bound and arthritis sufferers.

Neck roll: Look to the right, then roll your head forward, as if you are trying to touch your chin to your chest. Keep rolling until you are looking over your left shoulder. Repeat in the other direction.

Shoulder lift: Relieve tension in the neck by lifting the shoulders toward the ears, then dropping them as low as they will go. Repeat 10 times.

Eat healthy foods. You should never skip meals. Take time out for lunch no matter how busy you are.

Carry nutritious snacks to the office, or even the shopping mall. A nutritionally balanced diet is important. For example, researchers have found that even small deficiencies of thiamin, a B-complex vitamin, can cause anxiety symptoms. Pantothenic acid, another B-complex vitamin, is critical during times of stress.

Avoid caffeine, alcohol, and large amounts of sweets, which can aggravate symptoms of stress.

Don't let others get you down. Choose positive friends whoa re not worriers. Friends who constantly put you down or talk gloomily about life will increase your anxiety.

Ask a good friend to help you talk out a problem and get it off your chest. A long-distance call to an old pal can be great therapy.

Forgive others instead of holding grudges. Relax your standards – for yourself and others. Perfectionism is not the way to happiness. Become more flexible.

Communicate clearly with your co-workers and boss. Ask questions. Repeat instructions that you are given. Clarifying directions at the start of a project can save hours later straightening out misunderstandings.

Be truthful with others. Lies and deception lead to stress that always takes it toll.

Be optimistic. Count your blessings, especially when everything seems to go wrong. Believe that most people are doing the best that they can.

Don't blow problems out of proportion. Live by a philosophy of life that whittles problems down to size. The maxim, "Live one day at a time," has helped millions.

Plan your time wisely. And realistically. For example, don't schedule back-to-back meetings with tight travel time. Remember to leave room for unanticipated events – both negative and positive. Be flexible about rearranging your agenda.

Get up 15 minutes early in the morning. Allow an extra 15 minutes to get to all appointments.

Avoid procrastination. Whatever needs doing, do it now. Schedule unpleasant tasks early, so that you won't have to worry about them for the rest of the day.

Keep an appointment book. Don't rely on your memory.

Do one thing at a time. Focus your attention on the person talking to you or the job at hand, instead of worrying about other things. This also reduces mistakes-which lead to more anxiety.

Be prepared to wait. Carry a book to read in case of delays.

Say "no" to requests that stretch you to the limits.

Delegate. You don't have to do it all yourself. Break a job into separate tasks and assign them to people with the appropriate skills. Then leave them alone to do their work.

Prevent problems before they occur. This takes some planning.

If you are flying to another city for an important meeting, carry your presentation materials and dress suit on board the plane. Baggage does get lost.

Buy gas for the car before the tank is empty. Get regular oil changes and checkups.

Keep food staples on hand so you can fix a fast meal without going to the store.

Keep food, toilet paper and toiletries on hand so you never run out. The same goes for postage stamps, paper and envelopes.

Keep duplicate keys for home, car and office in secure locations.

Retreat to recharge your spirit. Schedule private time every day. You deserve it. Unplug the telephone and enjoy a quiet evening alone or with your family, or even 15 uninterrupted minutes in the shower or bathtub.

You may want to spend a few minutes writing your feelings out in a journal. It can help you find a new perspective and relieve hidden conflicts.

Here are more spirit rechargers:

Wear earplugs for instant peach anytime, anyplace.

Learn a meditation technique. Two methods: Observe your thoughts as they pass through your mind. Or, repeat a word or phrase with an uplifting meaning.

Practice progressive relaxation for 20 minutes twice a day to relive high blood pressure and other physiological responses to stress. Tighten and release each muscle group in turn, starting with the soles of the feet and slowly working up to the scalp.

Plan a weekend activity that is a change of pace. If your week is heavily scheduled, relax and enjoy noncompetitive activities. If you are never able to finish anything during the week, choose a project that you can complete in a few hours on Saturday or Sunday.

Take time out for a diversion in the middle of your workday. When the pressures of completing a project are too great, your productivity can drop. Take a walk or stop for lunch.

Savor life's little delights. Give yourself some physical pleasure to help your stress slip away.

Treat yourself to a professional massage, or trade massages with a loved one.

Give yourself permission to enjoy a move, watch a sports event, listen to music or read a book.

Savor a soothing cup of chamomile herb tea with a dollop of honey. Chamomile has long been used to relieve nervous tension.

Plan a day of beauty with a friend. Do each other's hair, or paint your nails and chat.

Create a simple steam facial at home by boiling water. Remove the pan from the stove. Cover your head with a large towel so that it creates a tent over the pot. Steam your face for five or 10 minutes. Add aromatic herbs to the water for a sensual touch.

Focus completely on any of the senses – hearing, seeing, eating or body movements – for a few minutes. Even washing your hands can become a sensual experience.

Use visualization and affirmation techniques. You can inoculate yourself against a situation you fear by going over the event in your mind. Imagine the scene in vivid detail and picture the best possible outcome.

You can also shrink an imagined fear down to size by picturing the worst possible results. Imagine describing this worst case to your best friend the next day and the sympathy you receive. Imagine telling a group of friends the next month, who share their similar experiences. Finally, imagine joking about your unpleasant experience with a complete stranger a year later. If you carry this exercise through to the end, your stress will become something to laugh about.

Replace negative self-talk with affirmations. The chatterbox in your mind is filled with gloom: You're too fat. . . you're too old. . .you'll never amount to anything. Like the little engine that could, nourish your mind with a constant stream of "I know I can."

Get enough sleep. Determine how much sleep you require for optimum performance. Sleep deprivation aggravates the body's responses to stress. Consider setting an alarm clock to remind yourself that it is time to go to bed.

Strive for your dreams. Plan ahead to meet your most cherished goals in life.

Time management experts emphasize the importance of writing down your important goals.

Break big projects down into a series of small steps that you can work on every day. Want to change jobs? Make on phone call contact today. Is writing a book your dream? Commit to writing one page a day.

Knowing that you are striving toward your dreams relieves frustrations that mount when you feel stuck in a rut of endless responsibilities that seem to lead nowhere.

Even if you only use these last 12 keys to stress relief, you can become a happier, healthier person, a more efficient worker and a better friend to others. Keep a notebook as new ideas come to you through your reading and your own creativity. The most important key is your decision to take time for yourself and to simplify your life whenever possible.

THE LITTLE TEST

Alpha

SCORE

Below 20 - How long have you had this problem with telling the truth?

Below 40 - You are super cool but perhaps should try to introduce some interest and excitement into your life. Get a hobby that you are passionate about!

40 -50 You are as cool as a cucumber and should serve as a role model for those around you.

51 -70 There are some issues you should address in your life but you have normal stress levels and cope well with mild extra stress.

71 - 90 Your stress levels are slightly elevated. You can choose to address them now or leave them to get worse.

91-110 Your stress levels are elevated beyond normal. You should attempt to modify or alter the way you deal with stress or your health may suffer.

111-130 You are excessively stressed. You need to take action now to modify or alter the way you cope with stress. You may of course already know what your

individual stressors are and therefore know
the solution to your stress.

130+ You are super stressed and possibly heading for disaster. If you have symptoms such as palpitations, shortness of breath, panic attacks, fainting, excessive sweating, IBS, food intolerance or any known medical condition you should see a medical practitioner to eliminate the possibility of physical ailments or conditions.

Resources: http://www.weightloss-expert-group.com

How To Stop Worrying And Start Living By Dale Carnegie

****

BOOK FOUR: YOGIC BREATHING!

■■

YOGA Science of Breath

A Complete Manual of THE ORIENTAL BREATHING PHILOSOPHY of Physical, Mental, Psychic and Spiritual Development.

By YOGI RAMACHARAKA

(I would like to thank YOGI RAMACHARAKA for this material)
Dr.Morgan..

INDEX.

CHAPTER

The Last Weight-loss Program You Will Ever Need

The Last Weight-loss Program You Will Ever Need

CHAPTER I.

SALUTATIONS.

The Western student is apt to be somewhat confused in his ideas regarding the Yogis and their philosophy and practice. Travelers to India have written great tales about the hordes of fakirs, mendicants and mountebanks who infest the great roads of India and the streets of its cities, and who impudently claim the title "Yogi." The Western student is scarcely to be blamed for thinking of the typical Yogi as an emaciated, fanatical, dirty, ignorant Hindu, who either sits in a fixed posture until his body becomes ossified, or else holds his arm up in the air until it becomes stiff and withered and forever after remains in that position, or perhaps clenches his fist and holds it tight until his fingernails grow through the palms of his hands. That these people exist is true, but their claim to the title "Yogi" seems as absurd to the true Yogi as does the claim to the title "Doctor" on the part of the man who pares one's corns seem to the eminent surgeon, or as does the title of "Professor," as assumed by the street corner vendor of worm medicine, seem to the President of Harvard or Yale.

There have been for ages past in India and other Oriental countries men who devoted their time and attention to the development of Man, physically, mentally and spiritually. The experience of generations of earnest seekers has been handed down for centuries from teacher to pupil, and gradually a definite Yogi science was built up. To these investigations and teachings was finally applied the term "Yogi," from the Sanscrit word "Yug," meaning "to join." From the same source comes the English word "yoke," with a similar meaning. Its use in connection with these teachings is difficult to trace, different authorities giving different explanations, but probably the most ingenious is that which holds that it is intended as the Hindu equivalent for the idea conveyed by the English phrase, "getting into harness," or "yoking up," as the Yogi undoubtedly "gets into harness" in his work of controlling the body and mind by the Will.

Yoga is divided into several branches, ranging from that which teaches the control of the body, to that which teaches the attainment of the highest spiritual development. In the work we will not go into the higher phases of the subject, except when the "Science of Breath" touches upon the same. The "Science of Breath" touches Yoga at many points, and although chiefly concerned with the development and control of the physical, has also its psychic side, and even enters the field of spiritual development.

The Last Weight-loss Program You Will Ever Need

In India there are great schools of Yoga, comprising thousands of the leading minds of that great country. The Yoga philosophy is the rule of life for many people. The pure Yogi teachings, however, are given only to the few, the masses being satisfied with the crumbs which fall from the tables of the educated classes, the Oriental custom in this respect being opposed to that of the Western world. But Western ideas are beginning to have their effect even in the Orient, and teachings which were once given only to the few are now freely offered to any who are ready to receive them. The East and the West are growing closer together, and both are profiting by the close contact, each influencing the other.

The Hindu Yogis have always paid great attention to the Science of Breath, for reasons which will be apparent to the student who reads this book. Many Western writers have touched upon this phase of the Yogi teachings, but we believe that it has been reserved for the writer of this work to give to the Western student, in concise form and simple language, the underlying principles of the Yogi Science of Breath, together with many of the favorite Yogi breathing exercises and methods. We have given the Western idea as well as the Oriental, showing how one dovetails into the other. We have used the ordinary English terms, almost entirely, avoiding the Sanscrit terms, so confusing to the average Western reader.

The first part of the book is devoted to the physical phase of the Science of Breath; then the psychic and mental sides are considered, and finally the spiritual side is touched upon.

We may be pardoned if we express ourselves as pleased with our success in condensing so much Yogi lore into so few pages, and by the use of words and terms which may be understood by anyone. Our only fear is that its very simplicity may cause some to pass it by as unworthy of attention, while they pass on their way searching for something "deep," mysterious and non-understandable. However, the Western mind is eminently practical, and we know that it is only a question of a short time before it will recognize the practicability of this work.

We greet our students, with our most profound salaam, and bid them be seated for their first lessons in the Yogi Science of Breath.

CHAPTER II.

"BREATH IS LIFE."

Life is absolutely dependent upon the act of breathing. "Breath is Life."

Differ as they may upon details of theory and terminology, the Oriental and the Occidental agree upon these fundamental principles.

To breathe is to live, and without breath there is no life. Not only are the higher animals dependent upon breath for life and health, but even the lower forms of animal life must breathe to live, and plant life is likewise dependent upon the air for continued existence.

The infant draws in a long, deep breath, retains it for a moment to extract from it its life-giving properties, and then exhales it in a long wail, and lo! its life upon earth has begun. The old man gives a faint gasp, ceases to breathe, and life is over. From the first faint breath of the infant to the last gasp of the dying man, it is one long story of continued breathing. Life is but a series of breaths.

Breathing may be considered the most important of all of the functions of the body, for, indeed, all the other functions depend upon it. Man may exist some time without eating; a shorter time without drinking; but without breathing his existence may be measured by a few minutes.

And not only is Man dependent upon Breath for life, but he is largely dependent upon correct habits of breathing for continued vitality and freedom from disease. An intelligent control of our breathing power will lengthen our days upon earth by giving us increased vitality and powers of resistance, and, on the other hand, unintelligent and careless breathing will tend to shorten our days, by decreasing our vitality and laying us open to disease.

Man in his normal state had no need of instruction in breathing. Like the lower animal and the child, he breathed naturally and properly, as nature intended him to do, but civilization has changed him in this and other respects. He has contracted improper methods and attitudes of walking, standing and sitting, which have robbed him of his birthright of natural and correct breathing. He has paid a high price for civilization. The savage, to-day, breathes naturally, unless he has been contaminated by the habits of civilized man.

The percentage of civilized men who breathe correctly is quite small, and the result is shown in contracted chests and stooping shoulders, and the terrible increase in diseases of the respiratory organs, including that dread monster, Consumption, "the white scourge." Eminent authorities have stated that one generation of correct breathers would regenerate the race, and disease would be so rare as to be looked upon as a curiosity. Whether looked at from the standpoint of the Oriental or Occidental, the connection between correct breathing and health is readily seen and explained.

The Occidental teachings show that the physical health depends very materially upon correct breathing. The Oriental teachers not only admit that their Occidental brothers are right, but say that in addition to the physical benefit derived from correct habits of breathing, Man's mental power, happiness, self-control, clear-sightedness, morals, and even his spiritual growth may be increased by an understanding of the "Science of Breath." Whole schools of Oriental Philosophy have been founded upon this science, and this knowledge when grasped by the Western races, and by them put to the practical use which is their strong point, will work wonders among them. The theory of the East, wedded to the practice of the West, will produce worthy offspring.

This work will take up the Yogi "Science of Breath," which includes not only all that is known to the Western physiologist and hygienist, but the occult side of the subject as well. It not only points out the way to physical health along the lines of what Western scientists have termed "deep breathing," etc., but also goes into the less known phases of the subject, and shows how the Hindu Yogi controls his body, increasing his mental capacity, and develops the spiritual side of his nature by the "Science of Breath."

The Yogi practices exercises by which he attains control of his body, and is enabled to send to any organ or part an increased flow of vital force or "prana," thereby strengthening and invigorating the part or organ. He knows all that his Western scientific brother knows about the physiological effect of correct breathing, but he also knows that the air contains more than oxygen and hydrogen and nitrogen, and that something more is accomplished than the mere oxygenating of the blood. He knows something about "prana," of which his Western brother is ignorant, and he is fully aware of the nature and manner of handling that great principle of energy, and is fully informed as to its effect upon the human body and mind. He knows that by rhythmical breathing one may bring

himself into harmonious vibration with nature, and aid in the unfoldment of his latent powers. He knows that by controlled breathing he may not only cure disease in himself and others, but also practically do away with fear and worry and the baser emotions.

To teach these things is the object of this work. We will give in a few chapters concise explanations and instructions, which might be extended into volumes. We hope to awaken the minds of the Western world to the value of the Yogi "Science of Breath."

CHAPTER III.

THE EXOTERIC THEORY OF BREATH.

In this chapter we will give you briefly the theories of the Western scientific world regarding the functions of the respiratory organs, and the part in the human economy played by the breath. In subsequent chapters we will give the additional theories and ascertained facts of the Oriental school of thought and research. The Oriental accepts the theories and facts of his Western brothers (which have been known to him for centuries) and adds thereto much that the latter do not now accept, but which they will in due time "discover" and which, after renaming, they will present to the world as a great truth.

Before taking up the Western idea, it will perhaps be better to give a hasty general idea of the Organs of Respiration.

The Organs of Respiration consist of the lungs and the air passages leading to them. The lungs are two in number, and occupy the pleural chamber of the thorax, one en each side of the median line, being separated from each other by the heart, the greater blood vessels and the larger air tubes. Each lung is free in all directions, except at the root, which consists chiefly of the bronchi, arteries and veins connecting the lungs with the trachea and heart. The lungs are spongy and porous, and their tissues are very elastic. They are covered with a delicately constructed but strong sac, known as the pleural sac, one wall of which closely adheres to the lung, and the other to the inner wall of the chest, and which secretes a fluid which allows the inner surfaces of the walls to glide easily upon each other in the act of breathing.

The Air Passages consist of the interior of the nose, pharynx, larynx, windpipe or trachea, and the bronchial tubes. When we breathe, we draw in the air through the nose, in which it is warmed by contact with the mucous membrane, which is richly supplied with blood, and after it has passed through the pharynx and larynx it passes into the trachea or windpipe, which subdivides into numerous tubes called the bronchial tubes (bronchia), which in turn subdivide into and terminate in minute subdivisions in all the small air spaces in the lungs, of which the lungs contain millions. A writer has stated that if the air cells of the lungs were spread out over an unbroken surface, they would cover an area of fourteen thousand square feet.

The air is drawn into the lungs by the action of the diaphragm, a great, strong, flat, sheet-like muscle, stretched across the chest, separating the chest-box from the abdomen. The diaphragm's action is almost as automatic as that of the heart, although it may be transformed into a semi-voluntary muscle by an effort of the will. When it expands, it increases the size of the chest and lungs, and the air rushes into the vacuum thus created. When it relaxes the chest and lungs contract and the air is expelled from the lungs.

Now, before considering what happens to the air in the lungs, let us look a little into the matter of the circulation of the blood. The blood, as you know, is driven by the heart, through the arteries, into the capillaries, thus reaching every part of the body, which it vitalizes, nourishes and strengthens. It then returns by means of the capillaries by another route, the veins, to the heart, from whence it is drawn to the lungs.

The blood starts on its arterial journey, bright red and rich, laden with life-giving qualities and properties. It returns by the venous route, poor, blue and dull, being laden down with the waste matter of the system. It goes out like a fresh stream from the mountains; it returns as a stream of sewer water. This foul stream goes to the right auricle of the heart. When this auricle becomes filled, it contracts and forces the stream of blood through an opening in the right ventricle of the heart, which in turn sends it on to the lungs, where it is distributed by millions of hair-like blood vessels to the air cells of the lungs, of which we have spoken. Now, let us take up the story of the lungs at this point.

The foul stream of blood is now distributed among the millions of tiny air cells in the lungs. A breath of air is inhaled and the oxygen of the air comes in contact with the impure blood through the thin walls of the hair-like blood vessels of the lungs, which walls are thick enough to hold the blood, but thin enough to admit the oxygen to penetrate them. When the oxygen comes in contact with the blood, a form of combustion takes place, and the blood takes up oxygen and releases carbonic acid gas generated from the waste products and poisonous matter which has been gathered up by the blood from all parts of the system.

The blood thus purified and oxygenated is carried back to the heart, again rich, red and bright, and laden with life-giving properties and qualities. Upon reaching the left auricle of the heart, it is forced into the left ventricle, from whence it is again forced out through the arteries on its mission of life to all parts of the system. It is estimated that in a single day of twenty-four hours, 35,000 pints of blood traverse the capillaries of the lungs, the blood corpuscles passing in single file and being exposed to the oxygen of the air on both of their surfaces. When one considers the minute details of the process alluded to, he is lost in wonder and admiration at Nature's infinite care and intelligence.

It will be seen that unless fresh air in sufficient quantities reaches the lungs, the foul stream of venous blood cannot be purified, and consequently not only is the body thus robbed of nourishment, but the waste products which should have been destroyed are returned to the circulation and poison the system, and death ensues. Impure air acts in the same way, only in a lessened degree. It will also be seen that if one does not breathe in a sufficient quantity of air, the work of the blood cannot go on properly, and the result is that the body is insufficiently nourished and disease ensues, or a state of imperfect health is experienced. The blood of one who breathes improperly is, of course, of a bluish, dark color, lacking the rich redness of pure arterial blood. This often shows itself in a poor complexion. Proper breathing, and a consequent good circulation, results in a clear, bright complexion.

A little reflection will show the vital importance of correct breathing. If the blood is not fully purified by the regenerative process of the lungs, it returns to the arteries in an abnormal state, insufficiently purified and imperfectly cleansed of the impurities which it took up on its return journey. These impurities if returned to the system will certainly manifest in some form of disease, either in a form of blood disease or some disease resulting from impaired functioning of some insufficiently nourished organ or tissue.

The blood, when properly exposed to the air in the lungs, not only has its impurities consumed, and parts with its noxious carbonic acid gas, but it also takes up and absorbs a certain quantity of oxygen which it carries to all parts of the body, where it is needed in order that Nature may perform her processes properly. When the oxygen comes in contact with the blood, it unites with the hemoglobin of the blood and is carried to every cell, tissue, muscle and organ, which it invigorates and strengthens, replacing the worn out cells and tissue by new materials which Nature converts to her use. Arterial blood, properly exposed to the air, contains about 25 per cent of free oxygen.

Not only is every part vitalized by the oxygen, but the act of digestion depends materially upon a certain amount of oxygenation of the food, and this can be accomplished only by the oxygen in the blood coming in contact with the food and producing a certain form of combustion. It is therefore necessary that a proper supply of oxygen be taken through the lungs. This accounts for the fact that weak lungs and poor digestion are so often found together. To grasp the full significance of this statement, one must remember that the entire body receives nourishment from the food assimilated, and that imperfect assimilation always means an imperfectly nourished body. Even the lungs themselves depend upon the same source for nourishment, and if through imperfect breathing the assimilation becomes imperfect, and the lungs in turn become weakened, they are rendered still less able to perform their work properly, and so in turn the body becomes further weakened. Every particle of food and drink must be oxygenated before it can yield us the proper nourishment, and before the waste products of the system can be reduced to the proper condition to be eliminated from the system. Lack of sufficient oxygen means Imperfect nutrition, Imperfect elimination and imperfect health. Verily, "breath is life."

The combustion arising from the change in the waste products generates heat and equalizes the temperature of the body. Good breathers are not apt to "take cold," and they generally have plenty of good warm blood which enables them to resist the changes in the outer temperature.

In addition to the above-mentioned important processes the act of breathing gives exercise to the internal organs and muscles, which feature is generally overlooked by the Western writers on the subject, but which the Yogis fully appreciate.

In imperfect or shallow breathing, only a portion of the lung cells are brought into play, and a great portion of the lung capacity is lost, the system suffering in proportion to the amount of under-oxygenation. The lower animals, in their native state, breathe naturally, and primitive man undoubtedly did the same. The abnormal manner of living adopted by civilized man—the shadow that follows upon civilization—has robbed us of our natural habit of breathing, and the race has greatly suffered thereby. Han's only physical salvation is to "get back to Nature."

CHAPTER IV.

THE ESOTERIC THEORY OF BREATH.

The Science of Breath, like many other teachings, has its esoteric or inner phase, as well as its exoteric or external. The physiological phase may be termed the outer or exoteric side of the subject, and the phase which we will now consider may be termed its esoteric or inner side. Occultists, in all ages and lands, have always taught, usually secretly to a few followers, that there was to be found in the air a substance or principle from which all activity, vitality and life was derived. They differed in their terms and names for this force, as well as in the details of the theory, but the main principle is to be found in all occult teachings and philosophies, and has for centuries formed a portion of the teachings of the Oriental Yogis.

In order to avoid misconceptions arising from the various theories regarding this great principle, which theories are usually attached to some name given the principle, we, in this work, will speak of the principle as "Prana," this word being the Sanskrit term meaning "Absolute Energy." Many occult authorities teach that the principle which the Hindus term "Prana" is the universal principle of energy or force, and that all energy or force is derived from that principle, or, rather, is a particular form of manifestation of that principle. These theories do not concern us in the consideration of the subject matter of this work, and we will therefore confine ourselves to an understanding of prana as the principle of energy exhibited in all living things, which distinguishes them from a lifeless thing. We may consider it as the active principle of life—Vital Force, if you please.

It is found in all forms of life, from the amoeba to man—from the most elementary form of plant life to the highest form of animal life. Prana is all pervading. It is found in all things having life, and as the occult philosophy teaches that life is in all things—in every atom—the apparent lifelessness of some things being only a lesser degree of manifestation, we may understand their teachings that prana is everywhere, in everything. Prana must not be confounded with the Ego—that bit of Divine Spirit in every soul, around which clusters matter and energy. Prana is merely a form of energy used by the Ego in its material manifestation. When the Ego leaves the body, the prana, being no longer under its control, responds only to the orders of the individual atoms, or groups of atoms, forming the body, and as the body disintegrates and is resolved to its original elements, each atom takes with it sufficient prana to enable it to form new combinations, the unused prana returning to the great universal storehouse from which it came. With the

Ego in control, cohesion exists and the atoms are held together by the Will of the Ego.

Prana is the name by which we designate a universal principle, which principle is the essence of all motion, force or energy, whether manifested in gravitation, electricity, the revolution of the planets, and all forms of life, from the highest to the lowest. It may be called the soul of Force and Energy in all their forms, and that principle which, operating in a certain way, causes that form of activity which accompanies Life.

This great principle is in all forms of matter, and yet it is not matter. It is in the air, but it is not the air nor one of its chemical constituents. Animal and plant life breathe it in with the air, and yet if the air contained it not they would die even though they might be filled with air. It is taken up by the system along with the oxygen, and yet is not the oxygen. The Hebrew writer of the book of Genesis knew the difference between the atmospheric air and the mysterious and potent principle contained within it. He speaks of neshemet ruach chayim, which, translated, means "the breath of the spirit of life." In the Hebrew neshemet means the ordinary breath of atmospheric air, and chayim means life or lives, while the word ruach means the "spirit of life," which occultists claim is the same principle which we speak of as Prana.

Prana is in the atmospheric air, but it is also elsewhere, and it penetrates where the air cannot reach. The oxygen in the air plays an important part in sustaining animal life, and the carbon plays a similar part with plant life, but Prana has its own distinct part to play in the manifestation of life, aside from the physiological functions.

We are constantly inhaling the air charged with prana, and are as constantly extracting the latter from the air and appropriating it to our uses. Prana is found in its freest state in the atmospheric air, which when fresh is fairly charged with it, and we draw it to us more easily from the air than from any other source. In ordinary breathing we absorb and extract a normal supply of prana, but by controlled and regulated breathing (generally known as Yogi breathing) we are enabled to extract a greater supply, which is stored away in the brain and nerve centers, to be used when necessary. We may store away prana, just as the storage battery stores away electricity. The many powers attributed to advanced occultists is due largely to their knowledge of this fact and their intelligent use of this stored-up energy. The Yogis know that by certain forms of breathing they establish certain relations with the supply of prana and may draw on the same for what they require. Not only do they strengthen all parts of their body in this way, but the brain itself may receive increased energy from the same source, and latent faculties be developed and psychic powers attained. One who has mastered the science of storing away prana, either consciously or unconsciously, often radiates vitality and strength which is felt by those coming in contact with him, and such a person may impart this strength to others, and give them increased vitality and health. What is called "magnetic healing" is performed in this way, although many practitioners are not aware of the source of their power.

Western scientists have been dimly aware of this great principle with which the air is charged, but finding that they could find no chemical trace of it, or make it register an any of their instruments, they have generally treated the Oriental theory with disdain. They could not explain this principle, and so denied it. They seem, however, to recognize that the air in certain places possesses a greater amount of "something" and sick people are directed by their physicians to seek such places in hopes of regaining, lost health.

The oxygen in the air is appropriated by the blood and is made use of by the circulatory system. The prana in the air is appropriated by the nervous system, and is used in its work. And as the oxygenated blood is carried to all parts of the system, building up and replenishing, so is the prana carried to all parts of the nervous system, adding strength and vitality. If we think of prana as being the active principle of what we call "vitality," we will be able to form a much clearer idea of what an important part it plays in our lives. Just as is the oxygen in the blood used up by the wants of the system, so the supply of prana taken up by the nervous system is exhausted by our thinking, willing, acting, etc., and in consequence constant replenishing is necessary. Every thought, every act, every effort of the will, every motion of a muscle, uses up a certain amount of what we call nerve force, which is really a form of prana. To move a muscle the brain sends out an impulse over the nerves, and the muscle contracts, and so much prana is expended. When it is remembered that the greater portion of prana acquired by man comes to him from the air inhaled, the importance of proper breathing is readily understood.

CHAPTER V.

THE NERVOUS SYSTEM.

It will be noticed that the Western scientific theories regarding the breath confine themselves to the effects of the absorption of oxygen, and its use through the circulatory system, while the Yogi theory also takes into consideration the absorption of Prana, and its manifestation through the channels of the Nervous System. Before proceeding further, it may be as well to take a hasty glance at the Nervous System.

The Nervous System of man is divided into two great systems, viz., the Cerebro-Spinal System and the Sympathetic System. The Cerebro-Spinal System consists of all that part of the Nervous System contained within the cranial cavity and the spinal canal, viz., the brain and the spinal cord, together with the nerves which branch off from the same. This system presides over the functions of animal life known as volition, sensation, etc. The Sympathetic System includes all that part of the Nervous System located principally in the thoracic, abdominal and pelvic cavities, and which is distributed to the internal organs. It has control over the involuntary processes, such as growth, nutrition, etc.

The Cerebro-Spinal System attends to all the seeing, hearing, tasting, smelling, feeling, etc. It sets things in motion; it is used by the Ego to think—to manifest consciousness. It is the instrument with which the Ego communicates with the outside world. This system may be likened to a telephone system, with the brain as the central office, and the spinal column and nerves as cable and wires respectively.

The brain is a great mass of nerve tissue, and consists of three parts, viz., the Cerebrum or brain proper, which occupies the upper, front, middle and back portion of the skull; the Cerebellum, or "little brain," which fills the lower and back portion of the skull; and the Medulla Oblongata, which Is the broadened commencement of the spinal cord, lying before and in front of the Cerebellum.

The Cerebrum is the organ of that part of the mind which manifests itself in intellectual action. The Cerebellum regulates the movements of the voluntary muscles. The Medulla Oblongata is the upper enlarged end of the spinal cord, and from it and the Cerebrum branch forth the Cranial Nerves which reach to various parts of the head, to the organs of special sense, and to some of the thoracic and abdominal organs, and to the organs of respiration.

The Spinal Cord, or spinal marrow, fills the spinal canal in the vertebral column, or "backbone." It is a long mass of nerve tissue, branching off at the several vertebrae to nerves communicating with all parts of the body. The Spinal Cord is like a large telephone cable, and the emerging nerves are like the private wires connecting therewith.

The Sympathetic Nervous System consists of a double chain of Ganglia on the side of the Spinal column, and scattered ganglia in the head, neck, chest and abdomen. (A ganglion is a mass of nervous matter including nerve cells.) These ganglia are connected with each other by filaments, and are also connected with the Cerebro-Spinal System by motor and sensory nerves. From these ganglia numerous fibers branch out to the organs of the body, blood vessels, etc. At various points, the nerves meet together and form what are known as plexuses. The Sympathetic System practically controls the involuntary processes, such as circulation, respiration and digestion.

The power or force transmitted from the brain to all parts of the body by means of the nerves, is known to Western science as "nerve force," although the Yogi knows it to be a manifestation of Prana. In character and rapidity it resembles the electric current. It will be seen that without this "nerve force" the heart cannot beat; the blood cannot circulate; the lungs cannot breathe; the various organs cannot function; in fact the machinery of the body comes to a stop without it. Nay more, even the brain cannot think without Prana be present. When these facts are considered, the importance of the absorption of Prana must be evident to all, and the Science of Breath assumes an importance even greater than that accorded it by Western science.

The Yogi teachings go further than does Western science, in one important feature of the Nervous System. We allude to what Western science terms the "Solar Plexus," and which it considers as merely one of a series of certain matted nets of sympathetic nerves with their ganglia found in various parts of the body. Yogi science teaches that this Solar Plexus is really a most important part of the Nervous System, and that it is a form of brain, playing one of the principal parts in the human economy. Western science seems to be moving gradually towards a recognition of this fact which has been known to the Yogis of the East for centuries, and some recent Western writers have termed the Solar Plexus the "Abdominal Brain." The Solar Plexus is situated in the Epigastric region, just back of the "pit of the stomach" on either side of the spinal column. It is composed of white and gray brain matter, similar to that composing the other brains of man. It has control of the main internal organs of man, and plays a much more important part than is generally recognized. We will not go into the Yogi theory regarding the Solar Plexus, further than to say that they know it as the great central storehouse of Prana. Men have been known to be instantly killed by a severe blow over the Solar Plexus, and prize fighters recognize its vulnerability and frequently temporarily paralyze their opponents by a blow over this region.

The name "Solar" is well bestowed on this "brain," as it radiates strength and energy to all parts of the body, even the upper brains depending largely upon it as a storehouse of Prana. Sooner or later Western science will fully recognize the real function of the Solar Plexus, and will accord to it a far more important place then it now occupies in their text-books and teachings.

CHAPTER VI.

NOSTRIL-BREATHING VS. MOUTH-BREATHING.

One of the first lessons in the Yogi Science of Breath, Is to learn how to breathe through the nostrils, and to overcome the common practice of mouth-breathing.

The breathing mechanism of Man is so constructed that he may breathe either through the mouth or nasal tubes, but it is a matter of vital importance to him which method he follows, as one brings health and strength and the other disease and weakness.

It should not be necessary to state to the student that the proper method of breathing is to take the breath through the nostrils, but alas! the ignorance among civilized people regarding this simple matter is astounding. We find people in all walks of life habitually breathing through their mouths, and allowing their children to follow their horrible and disgusting example.

Many of the diseases to which civilized man is subject are undoubtedly caused by this common habit of mouth-breathing. Children permitted to breathe in this way grow up with impaired vitality and weakened constitutions, and in manhood and womanhood break down and become chronic invalids. The mother of the savage race does better, being evidently guided by her intuition. She seems to instinctively recognize that the nostrils are the proper channels for the conveyal of air to the lungs, and she trains her infant to close its little lips and breathe through the nose. She tips its head forward when it is asleep, which attitude closes the lips and makes nostril-breathing imperative. If our civilized mothers were to adopt the same plan, it would work a great good for the race.

Many contagious diseases are contracted by the disgusting habit of mouth-breathing, and many cases of cold and catarrhal affections are also attributable to the same cause. Many persons who, for the sake of appearances, keep their mouth closed during the day, persist in mouth-breathing at night and often contract disease in this way.

Carefully conducted scientific experiments have shown that soldiers and sailors who sleep with their mouths open are much more liable to contract contagious diseases than those who breathe properly through the nostrils. An instance is related in which small-pox became epidemic on a man-of-war in foreign parts, and every death which resulted was that of some sailor or marine who was a mouth-breather, not a single nostril-breather succumbing.

The organs of respiration have their only protective apparatus, filter, or dust-catcher, in the nostrils. When the breath is taken through the mouth, there is nothing from mouth to lungs to strain the air, or to catch the dust and other foreign matter in the air. From mouth to lungs the dirt or impure substance has a clear track, and the entire respiratory system is unprotected. And, moreover, such incorrect breathing admits cold air to the organs, thereby injuring them. Inflammation of the respiratory organs often results from the inhalation of cold air through the mouth. The man who breathes through the mouth at night, always awakens with a parched feeling in the mouth and a dryness in the throat. He is violating one of nature's laws, and is sowing the seeds of disease.

Once more, remember that the mouth affords no protection to the respiratory organs, and cold air, dust and impurities and germs readily enter by that door. On the other hand, the nostrils and nasal passages show evidence of the careful design of nature in this respect. The nostrils are two narrow, tortuous channels, containing numerous bristly hairs which serve the purpose of a filter or sieve to strain the air of its impurities, etc., which are expelled when the breath is exhaled. Not only do the nostrils serve this important purpose, but they also perform an important function in warming the air inhaled. The long narrow winding nostrils are filled with warm mucous membrane, which coming in contact with the inhaled air Warms it so that it can do no damage to the delicate organs of the throat, or to the lungs.

No animal, excepting man, sleeps with the mouth open or breathes through the mouth, and in fact it is believed that it is only civilized man who so perverts nature's functions, as the savage and barbarian races almost invariably breathe correctly. It is probable that this unnatural habit among civilized men has been acquired through unnatural methods of living, enervating luxuries and excessive warmth.

The refining, filtering and straining apparatus of the nostrils renders the air fit to reach the delicate organs of the throat and the lungs, and the air is not fit to so reach these organs until it has passed through nature's refining process. The impurities which are stopped and retained by the sieves and mucous membrane of the nostrils, are thrown out again by the expelled breath, in exhalation, and in case they have accumulated too rapidly or have managed to escape through the sieves and have penetrated forbidden regions, nature protects us by producing a sneeze which violently ejects the intruder.

The air, when it enters the lungs is as different from the outside air, as is distilled water different from the water of the cistern. The intricate purifying organization of the nostrils, arresting and holding the impure particles in the air, is as important as is the action of the mouth in stopping cherry-stones and fish-bones and preventing them from being carried on to the stomach. Man should no more breathe through his mouth than he would attempt to take food through his nose.

Another feature of mouth-breathing is that the nasal passages, being thus comparatively unused, consequently fail to keep themselves clean and clear, and become clogged up and unclean, and are apt to contract local diseases. Like abandoned roads that soon become filled with weeds and rubbish, unused nostrils become filled with impurities and foul matter.

One who habitually breathes through the nostrils is not likely to be troubled with clogged or stuffy nostrils, but for the benefit of those who have been more or less addicted to the unnatural mouth-breathing, and who wish to acquire the natural and rational method, it may perhaps be well to add a few words regarding the way to keep their nostrils clean and free from impurities.

A favorite Oriental method is to snuff a little water up the nostrils allowing it to run down the passage into the throat, from thence it may be ejected through the mouth. Some Hindu yogis immerse the face in a bowl of water, and by a sort of suction draw in quite a quantity of water, but this latter method requires considerable practice, and the first mentioned method is equally efficacious, and much more easily performed.

Another good plan is to open the window and breathe freely, closing one nostril with the finger or thumb, sniffing up the air through the open nostril. Then repeat the process on the other nostril. Repeat several times, changing nostrils. This method will usually clear the nostrils of obstructions.

In case the trouble is caused by catarrh it is well to apply a little vaseline or camphor ice or similar preparation. Or sniff up a little witch-hazel extract once in a while, and you will notice a marked improvement. A little care and attention will result in the nostrils becoming clean and remaining so.

We have given considerable space to this subject of nostril-breathing, not only because of its great importance in its reference to health, but because nostril-breathing is a prerequisite to the practice of the breathing exercises to be given later in this book, and because nostril-breathing is one of the basic principles underlying the Yogi Science of Breath.

We urge upon the student the necessity of acquiring this method of breathing if he has it not, and caution him against dismissing this phase of the subject as unimportant.

CHAPTER VII.

FOUR METHODS OF RESPIRATION.

In the consideration of the question of respiration, we must begin by considering the mechanical arrangements whereby the respiratory movements are effected. The mechanics of respiration manifest through
(1) the elastic movements of the lungs, and (2) the activities of the sides and bottom of the thoracic cavity in which the lungs are contained. The thorax is that portion of the trunk between the neck and the abdomen, the cavity of which (known as the thoracic cavity) is occupied mainly by the lungs and heart. It is bounded by the spinal column, the ribs with their cartilages, the breastbone, and below by the diaphragm. It is generally spoken of as "the chest." It has been compared to a completely shut, conical box, the small end of which Is turned upward, the back of the box being formed by the spinal column, the front by the breastbone and the sides by the ribs.

(2)The ribs are twenty-four in number, twelve on each side, and emerge from each side of the spinal column. The upper seven pair are known as "true ribs," being fastened to the breastbone direct, while the lower five pairs are called (false ribs) or "floating ribs," because they are not so fastened, the upper two of them being fastened by cartilage to the other ribs, the remainder having no cartilages, their forward ends being free.

The ribs are moved in respiration by two superficial muscular layers, known as the intercostal muscles. The diaphragm, the muscular partition before alluded to, separates the chest box from the abdominal cavity.

In the act of inhalation the muscles expand the lungs so that a vacuum is created and the air rushes in in accordance with the well known law of physics. Everything depends upon the muscles concerned in the process of respiration, which we may as, for convenience, term the "respiratory muscles." Without the aid of these muscles the lungs cannot expand, and upon the proper use and control of these muscles the Science of Breath largely depends. The proper control of these muscles will result in the ability to attain the maximum degree of lung expansion, and the greatest amount of the life giving properties of the air into the system.

The Yogis classify Respiration into four general methods, viz:

(1) High Breathing.
(2) Mid Breathing.
(3) Low Breathing.
(4) Yogi Complete Breathing.

We will give a general idea of the first three methods, and a more extended treatment of the fourth method, upon which the Yogi Science of Breath is largely based.

(1)   HIGH BREATHING.

This form of breathing is known to the Western world as Cardiovascular Breathing, or Collarbone Breathing. One breathing in this way elevates the ribs and raises the collarbone and shoulders, at the same time drawing in the abdomen and pushing its contents up against the diaphragm, which in turn is raised.

The upper part of the chest and lungs, which is the smallest, is used, and consequently but a minimum amount of air enters the lungs. In addition to this, the diaphragm being raised, there can be no expansion in that direction. A study of the anatomy of the chest will convince any student that in this way a maximum amount of effort is used to obtain a minimum amount of benefit.

High Breathing is probably the worst form of breathing known to man and requires the greatest expenditure of energy with the smallest amount of benefit. It is an energy-wasting, poor-returns plan. It is quite common among the Western races, many women being addicted to It, and even singers, clergymen, lawyers and others, who should know better, using it ignorantly.

Many diseases of the vocal organs and organs of respiration may be directly traced to this barbarous method of breathing, and the straining of delicate organs caused by this method, often results in the harsh, disagreeable voices heard on all sides. Many persons who breathe In this way become addicted to the disgusting practice of "mouth-breathing" described in a preceding chapter.

If the student has any doubts about what has been said regarding this form of breathing, let him try the experiment of expelling all the air from his lungs, then standing erect, with hands at sides, let him raise the shoulders and collar-bone and inhale. He will find that the amount of air inhaled far below normal. Then let him inhale a full breath, after dropping the shoulders and collar-bone, and he will receive an object lesson in breathing which he will be apt to remember much longer than he would any words, printed or spoken.

(2)   MID BREATHING.

This method of respiration is known to Western students as Rib Breathing, or Inter-Costal Breathing, and while less objectionable than High Breathing, is far inferior to either Low Breathing or to the Yogi Complete Breath. In Mid Breathing the diaphragm is pushed upward, and the abdomen drawn in. The ribs are raised somewhat, and the chest is partially expanded. It is quite common among men who have made no study of the subject. As there are two better methods known, we give it only passing notice, and that principally to call your attention to its short-comings.

(2) LOW BREATHING.

This form of respiration is far better than either of the two preceding forms: and of recent years many Western writers have extolled its merits, and have exploited it under the names of "Abdominal Breathing," "Deep Breathing," "Diaphragmatic Breathing," etc., etc., and much good has been accomplished by the attention of the public having been directed to the subject, and many having been Induced to substitute it for the interior and injurious methods above alluded to. Many "systems" of breathing have been built around Low Breathing, and students have paid high prices to learn the new (?) systems. But, as we have said, much good has resulted, and after all the students who paid high prices to learn revamped old systems undoubtedly got their money's worth if they were Induced to discard the old methods of High Breathing and Low Breathing.

Although many Western authorities write and speak of this method as the best known form of breathing, the Yogis know it to be but a part of a system which they have used for centuries and which they know as "The Complete Breath." It must be admitted, however, that one must be acquainted with the principles of Low Breathing before he can grasp the idea of Complete Breathing.

Let us again consider the diaphragm. What is it? We have seen that it is the great partition muscle, which separates the chest and its contents from the abdomen and its contents. When at rest it presents a concave surface to the abdomen. That is, the diaphragm as viewed from the abdomen would seem like the sky as viewed from the earth—the interior of an arched surface. Consequently the side of the diaphragm toward the chest organs is like a protruding rounded surface—like a hill. When the diaphragm is brought into use the hill formation is lowered and the diaphragm presses upon the abdominal organs and forces out the abdomen.

In Low Breathing, the lungs are given freer play than in the methods already mentioned, and consequently more air is inhaled. This fact has led the majority of Western writers to speak and write of Low Breathing (which they call Abdominal Breathing) as the highest and best method known to science. But the Oriental Yogi has long known of a better method, and some few Western writers have also recognized this fact. The trouble with all methods of breathing, other than "Yogi Complete Breathing" is that in none of these methods do the lungs become filled with air—at the best only a portion of the lung space is filled, even in Low Breathing. High Breathing fills only the upper portion of the lungs. Mid Breathing fills only the middle and a portion of the upper parts. Low Breathing fills only the lower and middle parts. It is evident that any method that fills the entire lung space must be far preferable to those filling only certain parts Any method which will fill the entire lung space must be the greatest value to Man in the way of allowing him to absorb the greatest quantity of oxygen and to store away the greatest amount of prana. The Complete Breath is known to the Yogis to be the best method of respiration known to science.

 THE YOGI COMPLETE BREATH.

Yogi Complete Breathing includes all the good points of High Breathing, Mid Breathing and Low Breathing, with the objectionable features of each eliminated. It brings into play the entire respiratory apparatus, every part of the lungs, every air-cell, every respiratory muscle. The entire respiratory organism responds to this method of breathing, and the maximum amount of benefit is derived from the minimum expenditure of energy. The chest cavity is increased to its normal limits in all directions and every part of the machinery performs its natural work and functions.

One of the most important features of this method of breathing is the fact that the respiratory muscles are fully called into play, whereas in the other forms of breathing only a portion of these muscles are so used. In Complete Breathing, among other muscles, those controlling the ribs are actively used, which increases the space in which the lungs may expand, and also gives the proper support to the organs when needed, Nature availing herself of the perfection of the principle of leverage in this process. Certain muscles hold the lower ribs firmly in position, while other muscles bend them outward.

Then again, in this method, the diaphragm is under perfect control and is able to perform its functions properly, and in such manner as to yield the maximum degree of service.

In the rib-action, above alluded to, the lower ribs are controlled by the diaphragm which draws them slightly downward, while other muscles hold them in place and the intercostal muscles force them outward, which combined action increases the mid-chest cavity to its maximum. In addition to this muscular action, the upper ribs are also lifted and forced outward by the intercostal muscles, which increases the capacity of the upper chest to its fullest extent.

If you have studied the special features of the four given methods of breathing, you will at once see that the Complete Breath comprises all the advantageous features of the three other methods, plus the reciprocal advantages accruing from the combined action of the high-chest, mid-chest, and diaphragmatic regions, and the normal rhythm thus obtained.

In our next chapter, we will take up the Complete Breath in practice, and will give full directions for the acquirement of this superior method of breathing, with exercises, etc.

CHAPTER VIII.

 HOW TO ACQUIRE THE YOGI COMPLETE BREATH.

The Yogi Complete Breath is the fundamental breath of the entire Yogi Science of Breath, and the student must fully acquaint himself with it, and master it perfectly before he can hope to obtain results from the other forms of breath-mentioned and given in this book. He should not be content with half-learning it, but should go to work in earnest until it becomes his natural method of breathing. This will require work, time and patience, but without these things nothing is ever accomplished. There is no royal road to the Science of Breath, and the student must be prepared to practice and study in earnest if he expect to receive results. The results obtained by a complete mastery of the Science of Breath are great, and no one who has attained them would willingly go back to the old methods, and he will tell his friends that he considers himself amply repaid for all his work. We say these things now, that you may fully understand the necessity and importance of mastering this fundamental method of Yogi Breathing, instead of passing it by and trying some of the attractive looking variations given later on in this book. Again, we say to you: Start right, and right results will follow; but neglect your foundations and your entire building will topple over sooner or later.

Perhaps the better way to teach you how to develop the Yogi Complete Breath, would be to give you simple directions regarding the breath itself, and then follow up the same with general remarks concerning it, and then later on giving exercises for developing the chest, muscles and lungs which have been allowed to remain in an undeveloped condition by imperfect methods of breathing. Right here we wish to say that this Complete Breath is not a forced or abnormal thing, but on the contrary is a going back to first principles—a return to Nature. The healthy adult savage and the healthy infant of civilization both breathe in this manner, but civilized man has adopted unnatural methods of living, clothing, etc., and has lost his birthright. And we wish to remind the reader that the Complete Breath does not necessarily call for the complete filling of the lungs at every inhalation. One may inhale the average amount of air, using the Complete Breathing Method and distributing the air inhaled, be the quantity large or small, to all parts of the lungs. But one should inhale a series of full Complete Breaths several times a day, whenever opportunity offers, in order to keep the system in good order and condition.

The following simple exercise will give you a clear idea of what the Complete Breath is:

(1) Stand or sit erect. Breathing through the nostrils, inhale steadily, first filling the lower part of the lungs, which is accomplished by bringing into play the diaphragm, which descending exerts a gentle pressure on the abdominal organs, pushing forward the front walls of the abdomen. Then fill the middle part of the lungs, pushing out the lower ribs, breast-bone and chest. Then fill the higher portion of the lungs, protruding the upper chest, thus lifting the chest, including the upper six or seven pairs of ribs. In the final movement, the lower part of the abdomen will be slightly drawn in, which movement gives the lungs a support and also helps to fill the highest part of the lungs.

At first reading it may appear that this breath consists of three distinct movements. This, however, is not the correct idea. The inhalation is continuous, the entire chest cavity from the lowered diaphragm to the highest point of the chest in the region of the collar-bone, being expanded with a uniform movement. Avoid a jerky series of inhalations, and strive to attain a steady continuous action. Practice will soon overcome the tendency to divide the inhalation into three movements, and will result in a uniform continuous breath. You will be able to complete the inhalation in a couple of seconds after a little practice.

(2) Retain the breath a few seconds.

(3) Exhale quite slowly, holding the chest in a firm position, and having the abdomen in a little and lifting it upward slowly as the air leaves the lungs. When the air is entirely exhaled, relax the chest and abdomen. A little practice will render this part of the exercise easy, and the movement once acquired will be afterwards performed almost automatically.

(4)

It will be seen that by this method of breathing all parts of the respiratory apparatus is brought into action, and all parts of the lungs, including the most remote air cells, are exercised. The chest cavity is expanded in all directions. You will also notice that the Complete Breath is really a combination of Low, Mid and High Breaths, succeeding each other rapidly in the order given, in such a manner as to form one uniform, continuous, complete breath.

You will find it quite a help to you if you will practice this breath before a large mirror, placing the hands lightly over the abdomen so that you may feel the movements. At the end of the inhalation, it is well to occasionally slightly elevate the shoulders, thus raising the collarbone and allowing the air to pass freely into the small upper lobe of the right lung, which place is sometimes the breeding place of tuberculosis.

At the beginning of practice, you may have more or less trouble in acquiring the Complete Breath, but a little practice will make perfect, and when you have once acquired it you will never willingly return to the old methods.

CHAPTER IX.

PHYSIOLOGICAL EFFECT OF THE COMPLETE BREATH.

Scarcely too much can be said of the advantages attending the practice of the Complete Breath. And yet the student who has carefully read the foregoing pages should scarcely need to have pointed out to him such advantages.

The practice of the Complete Breath will make any man or woman immune to Consumption and other pulmonary troubles, and will do away with all liability to contract "colds," as well as bronchial and similar weaknesses. Consumption is due principally to lowered vitality attributable to an insufficient amount of air being inhaled. The impairment of vitality renders the system open to attacks from disease germs. Imperfect breathing allows a considerable part of the lungs to remain inactive, and such portions offer an inviting field for bacilli, which invading the weakened tissue soon produce havoc. Good healthy lung tissue will resist the germs, and the only way to have good healthy lung tissue is to use the lungs properly.

Consumptives are nearly all narrow-chested. What does this mean? Simply that these people were addicted to improper habits of breathing, and consequently their chests failed to develop and expand. The man who practices the Complete Breath will have a full broad chest, end the narrow-chested man may develop his chest to normal proportions if he will but adopt this mode of breathing. Such people must develop their chest cavities if they value their lives. Colds may often be prevented by practicing a little vigorous Complete Breathing whenever you feel that you are being unduly exposed. When chilled, breathe vigorously a few minutes, and you will feel a glow all over your body. Most colds can be cured by Complete Breathing and partial fasting for a day.

The quality of the blood depends largely upon its proper oxygenation in the lungs, and if it is under-oxygenated it becomes poor in quality and laden with all sorts of impurities, and the system suffers from lack of nourishment, and often becomes actually poisoned by the waste products remaining uneliminated in the blood. As the entire body, every organ and every part, is dependent upon the blood for nourishment, impure blood must have a serious effect upon the entire system. The remedy is plain—practice the Yogi Complete Breath.

The stomach and other organs of nutrition suffer much from improper breathing. Not only are they ill nourished by reason of the lack of oxygen, but as the food must absorb oxygen from the blood and become oxygenated before it can be digested and assimilated, it is readily seen how digestion and assimilation is impaired by incorrect breathing. And when assimilation is not normal, the system receives less and less nourishment, the appetite fails, bodily vigor decreases, and energy diminishes, and the man withers and declines. All from the lack of proper breathing.

Even the nervous system suffers from improper breathing, inasmuch as the brain, the spinal cord, the nerve centers, and the nerves themselves, when improperly nourished by means of the blood, become poor and inefficient instruments for generating, storing and transmitting the nerve currents. And improperly nourished they will become if sufficient oxygen is not absorbed through the lungs. There is another aspect of the case whereby the nerve currents themselves, or rather the force from which the nerve currents spring, becomes lessened from want of proper breathing, but this belongs to another phase of the subject which is treated of in other chapters of this book, and our purpose here is to direct your attention to the fact that the mechanism of the nervous system is rendered inefficient as an instrument for conveying nerve force, as the indirect result of a lack of proper breathing.

The effect of the reproductive organs upon the general health is too well known to be discussed at length here, but we may be permitted to say that with the reproductive organs in a weakened condition the entire system feels the reflex action and suffers sympathetically. The Complete Breath produces a rhythm which is Nature's own plan for keeping this important part of the system in normal condition, and, from the first, it will be noticed that the reproductive functions are strengthened and vitalized, thus, by sympathetic reflex action, giving tone to the whole system. By this, we do not mean that the lower sex impulses will be aroused; far from it.

The Yogis are advocates of continence and chastity, and have learned to control the animal passions. But sexual control does not mean sexual weakness, and the Yogi teachings are that the man or woman whose reproductive organism is normal and healthy, will have a stronger will with which to control himself or herself. The Yogi believes that much of the perversion of this wonderful part of the system comes from a lack of normal health, and results from a morbid rather than a normal condition of these organs. A little careful consideration of this question will prove that the Yogi teachings are right. This is not the place to discuss the subject fully, but the Yogis know that sex-energy may be conserved and used for the development of the body and mind of the individual, instead of being dissipated in unnatural excesses as is the wont of so many uninformed people. By special request we will give in this book one of the favorite Yogi exercises for this purpose. But whether or not the student wishes to adopt the Yogi theories of continence and clean-living, he or she will find that the Complete Breath will do more to restore health to this part of the system than anything else ever tried. Remember, now, we mean normal health, not undue development. The sensualist will find that normal means a lessening of desire rather than an increase; the weakened man or woman will find a toning up and a relief from the weakness which has heretofore depressed him or her. We do not wish to be misunderstood or misquoted on this subject. The Yogis' ideal is a body strong in all its parts, under the control of a masterful and developed Will, animated by high ideals.

In the practice of the Complete Breath, during inhalation, the diaphragm contracts and exerts a gentle pressure upon the liver, stomach and other organs, which in connection with the rhythm of the lungs acts as a gentle massage of these organs and stimulates their actions, and encourages normal functioning. Each inhalation aids in this internal exercise, and assists in causing a normal circulation to the organs of nutrition and elimination. In High or Mid Breathing the organs lose the benefit accruing from this internal massage.

The Western world is paying much attention to Physical Culture just now, which is a good thing. But in their enthusiasm they must not forget that the exercise of the external muscles is not everything. The internal organs also need exercise, and Nature's plan for this exercise is proper breathing. The diaphragm is Nature's principal instrument for this internal exercise. Its motion vibrates the important organs of nutrition and elimination, and massages and kneads them at each inhalation and exhalation, forcing blood into them, and then squeezing it out, and imparting a general tone to the organs. Any organ or part of the body which is not exercised gradually atrophies and refuses to function properly, and lack of the internal exercise afforded by the diaphragmatic action leads to diseased organs. The Complete Breath gives the proper motion to the diaphragm, as well as exercising the middle and upper chest. It is indeed "complete" in its action.

From the standpoint of Western physiology alone, without reference to the Oriental philosophies and science, this Yogi system of Complete Breathing is of vital importance to every man, woman and child who wishes to acquire health and keep it. Its very simplicity keeps thousands from seriously considering it, while they spend fortunes in seeking health through complicated and expensive "systems." Health knocks at their door and they answer not. Verily the stone which the builders reject is the real cornerstone of the Temple of Health.

CHAPTER X.

A FEW BITS OF YOGI LORE.

We give below three forms of breath, quite popular among the Yogis. The first is the well-known Yogi Cleansing Breath, to which is attributed much of the great lung endurance found among the Yogis. They usually finish up a breathing exercise with this Cleansing Breath, and we have followed this plan in this book. We also give the Yogi Nerve Vitalizing Exercise, which has been handed down among them for ages, and which has never been improved on by Western teachers of Physical Culture, although some of them have "borrowed" it from teachers of Yoga. We also give the Yogi Vocal Breath, which accounts largely for the melodious, vibrant voices of the better class of the Oriental Yogis. We feel that if this book contained nothing more than these three exercises, it would be invaluable to the Western student. Take these exercises as a gift from your Eastern brothers and put them into practice.

THE YOGI CLEANSING BREATH.

The Yogis have a favorite form of breathing which they practice when they feel the necessity of ventilating and cleansing the lungs. They conclude many of their other breathing exercises with this breath, and we have followed this practice in this book. This Cleansing Breath ventilates and cleanses the lungs, stimulates the cells and gives a general tone to the respiratory organs, and is conducive to their general healthy condition. Besides this effect, it is found to greatly refresh the entire system. Speakers, singers, etc., will find this breath especially restful, after having tired the respiratory organs.

   (1) Inhale a complete breath.
   (2) Retain the air a few seconds.
   (3) Pucker up the lips as if for a whistle (but do not swell out the cheeks), then exhale a little air through the opening, with considerable vigor. Then stop for a moment, retaining the air, and then exhale a little more air. Repeat until the air is completely exhaled. Remember that considerable vigor is to be used in exhaling the air through the opening in the lips.

This breath will be found quite refreshing when one is tired and generally "used up." A trial will convince the student of its merits. This exercise should be practiced until it can be performed naturally and easily, as it is used to finish up a number of other exercises given in this book, and it should be thoroughly understood.

THE YOGI NERVE VITALIZING BREATH.

This is an exercise well known to the Yogis, who consider it one of the strongest nerve stimulants and invigorants known to man. Its purpose is to stimulate the Nervous System, develop nerve force, energy and vitality. This exercise brings a stimulating pressure to bear on important nerve centers, which in turn stimulate and energize the entire nervous system, and send an increased flow of nerve force to all parts of the body.

(1) Stand erect.
(2) Inhale a Complete Breath, and retain same.
(3) Extend the arms straight in front of you, letting them be somewhat limp and relaxed, with only sufficient nerve force to hold them out.
(4) Slowly draw the hands back toward the shoulders, gradually contracting the muscles and putting force into them, so that when they reach the shoulders the fists will be so tightly clenched that a tremulous motion is felt.
(5) Then, keeping the muscles tense, push the fists slowly out, and then draw them back rapidly (still tense) several times.
(6) Exhale vigorously through the mouth.
(7) Practice the Cleansing Breath.

The efficiency of this exercise depends greatly upon the speed of the drawing back of the fists, and the tension of the muscles, and, of course, upon the full lungs. This exercise must be tried to be appreciated. It is without equal as a "bracer," as our Western friends put it.

THE YOGI VOCAL BREATH.

The Yogis have a form of breathing to develop the voice. They are noted for their wonderful voices, which are strong, smooth and clear, and have a wonderful trumpet-like carrying power. They have practiced this particular form of breathing exercise which has resulted in rendering their voices soft, beautiful and flexible, imparting to it that indescribable, peculiar floating quality, combined with great power. The exercise given below will in time impart the above-mentioned qualities, or the Yogi Voice, to the student who practices it faithfully. It is to be understood, of course, that this form of breath is to be used only as an occasional exercise, and not as a regular form of breathing.

(1) Inhale a Complete Breath very slowly, but steadily, through the nostrils, taking as much time as possible in the inhalation.
(2) Retain for a few seconds.
(3) Expel the air vigorously in one great breath, through the wide opened mouth.
(4) Rest the lungs by the Cleansing Breath.

Without going deeply into the Yogi theories of sound-production in speaking and singing, we wish to say that experience has taught them that the timbre, quality and power of a voice depends not alone upon the vocal organs in the throat, but that the facial muscles, etc., have much to do with the matter. Some men with large chests produce but a poor tone, while others with comparatively small chests produce tones of amazing strength and quality. Here is an interesting experiment worth trying: Stand before a glass and pucker up your mouth and whistle, and note the shape of your mouth and the general expression of your face. Then sing or speak as you do naturally, and see the difference. Then start to whistle again for a few seconds, and then, *without changing the position of your lips or face*, sing a few notes and notice what a vibrant, resonant, clear and beautiful tone is produced.

CHAPTER XI.

THE SEVEN YOGI DEVELOPING EXERCISES.

The following are the seven favorite exercises of the Yogis for developing the lungs, muscles, ligaments, air cells, etc. They are quite simple but marvelously effective. Do not let the simplicity of these exercises make you lose interest, for they are the result of careful experiments and practice on the part of the Yogis, and are the essence of numerous intricate and complicated exercises, the non-essential portions being eliminated and the essential features retained.

 (1)   THE RETAINED BREATH.

This is a very important exercise which tends to strengthen and develop the respiratory muscles as well as the lungs, and its frequent practice will also tend to expand the chest. The Yogis have found that an occasional holding of the breath, after the lungs have been filled with the Complete Breath, is very beneficial, not only to the respiratory organs but to the organs of nutrition, the nervous system and the blood itself. They have found that an occasional holding of the breath tends to purify the air which has remained in the lungs from former inhalations, and to more fully oxygenate the blood. They also know that the breath so retained gathers up all the waste matter, and when the breath is expelled it carries with it the effete matter of the system, and cleanses the lungs just as a purgative does the bowels. The Yogis recommend this exercise for various disorders of the stomach, liver and blood, and also find that it frequently relieves bad breath, which often arises from poorly ventilated lungs. We recommend students to pay considerable attention to this exercise, as it has great merits. The following directions will give you a clear idea of the exercise:

    (1) Stand erect.
    (2) Inhale a Complete Breath.

(3) Retain the air as long as you can comfortably.
(4) Exhale vigorously through the open mouth.
(5) Practice the Cleansing Breath.

At first you will be able to retain the breath only a short time, but a little practice will also show a great improvement. Time yourself with a watch if you wish to note your progress.

(2)   LUNG CELL STIMULATION.

This exercise is designed to stimulate the air cells in the lungs, but beginners must not overdo it, and in no case should it be indulged in too vigorously. Some may find a slight dizziness resulting from the first few trials, in which case let them walk around a little and discontinue the exercise for a while.

(1) Stand erect, with hands at sides.
(2) Breathe in very slowly and gradually.
(3) While inhaling, gently tap the chest with the finger tips, constantly changing position.
(4) When the lungs are filled, retain the breath and pat the chest with the palms of the hands.
(5) Practice the Cleansing Breath.

This exercise is very bracing and stimulating to the whole body, and is a well-known Yogi practice. Many of the air cells of the lungs become inactive by reason of incomplete breathing, and often become almost atrophied. One who has practiced imperfect breathing for years will find it not so easy to stimulate all these ill-used air cells into activity all at once by the Complete Breath, but this exercise will do much toward bringing about the desired result, and is worth study and practice.

(3)   RIB STRETCHING.

We have explained that the ribs are fastened by cartilages, which admit of considerable expansion. In proper breathing, the ribs play an important part, and it is well to occasionally give them a little special exercise in order to preserve their elasticity. Standing or sitting in unnatural positions, to which many of the Western people are addicted, is apt to render the ribs more or less stiff and inelastic, and this exercise will do much to overcome same.

(1) Stand erect.
(2) Place the hands one on each side of the body, as high up under the armpits as convenient, the thumbs reaching toward the back, the palms on the side of the chest and the fingers to the front over the breast.
(3) Inhale a Complete Breath.
(4) Retain the air for a short time.
(5) Then gently squeeze the sides, at the same time slowly exhaling.

(6) Practice the cleansing breath.

Use moderation in this exercise and do not overdo its

(4)   CHEST EXPANSION.

The chest is quite apt to be contracted from bending over one's work, etc. This exercise is very good for the purpose of restoring natural conditions and gaining chest expansion.

(1) Stand erect.
(2) Inhale a Complete Breath.
(3) Retain the air.
(4) Extend both arms forward and bring the two clenched fists together on a level with the shoulder.
(5) Then swing back the fists vigorously until the arms stand out straight sideways from the shoulders.
(6) Then bring back to Position 4, and swing to Position 5.
Repeat several times.

(7) Exhale vigorously through the opened mouth.
(8) Practice the Cleansing Breath.

Use moderation and do not overdo this exercise.

 (5)   WALKING EXERCISE.
(1) Walk with head up, chin drawn slightly in, shoulders back, and with measured tread.
(2) Inhale a Complete Breath, counting (mentally) 1, 2, 3, 4, 5, 6, 7, 8, one count to each step, making the inhalation extend over the eight counts.
(3) Exhale slowly through the nostrils, counting as before--1, 2, 3, 4, 5, 6, 7, 8--one count to a step.
(4) Rest between breaths, continuing walking and counting, I, 2, 3, 4, 5, 8, 7, 8, one count to a step.
(5) Repeat until you begin to feel tired. Then rest for a while, and resume at pleasure. Repeat several times a day.

Some Yogis vary this exercise by retaining the breath during a 1, 2, 3, 4, count, and then exhale in an eight-step count. Practice whichever plan seems most agreeable to you.

(6)   MORNING EXERCISE.
(1) Stand erect in a military attitude, head up, eyes front, shoulders back, knees stiff, hands at sides.

(2) Raise body slowly on toes, inhaling a Complete Breath, steadily and slowly.
(3) Retain the breath for a few seconds, maintaining the same position.
(4) Slowly sink to first position, at the same time slowly exhaling the air through the nostrils.
(5) Practice Cleansing Breath.
(6) Repeat several times, varying by using right leg alone, then left leg alone.

(7)   STIMULATING CIRCULATION.

(1) Stand erect.
(2) Inhale a Complete Breath and retain.
(3) Bend forward slightly and grasp a stick or cane steadily and firmly, and gradually exerting your entire strength upon the grasp.
(4) Relax the grasp, return to first position, and slowly exhale.
(5) Repeat several times.
(6) Finish with the Cleansing Breath.

This exercise may be performed without the use of a stick or cane, by grasping an imaginary cane, using the will to exert the pressure. The exercise is a favorite Yogi plan of stimulating the circulation by driving the arterial blood to the extremities, and drawing back the venous blood to the heart and lungs that it may take up the oxygen which has been inhaled with the air. In cases of poor circulation there is not enough blood in the lungs to absorb the increased amount of oxygen inhaled, and the system does not get the full benefit of the improved breathing.

In such cases, particularly, It Is well to practice this exercise, occasionally with the regular Complete Breathing exercise.

CHAPTER XII.

 SEVEN MINOR YOGI EXERCISES.

This chapter is composed of seven minor Yogi Breathing Exercises, bearing no special names, but each distinct and separate from the others and having a different purpose in view. Each student will find several of these exercises best adapted to the special requirements of his particular case. Although we have styled these exercises "minor exercises," they are quite valuable and useful, or they would not appear in this book. They give one a condensed course in "Physical Culture" and "Lung Development," and might readily be "padded out"

and elaborated into a small book on these subjects. They have, of course, an additional value, as Yogi Breathing forms a part of each exercise. Do not pass them by because they are marked "minor." Some one or more of these exercises may be just what you need. Try them and decide for yourself.

EXERCISE I.
(1) Stand erect with hands at sides.
(2) Inhale Complete Breath.
(3) Raise the arms slowly, keeping them rigid until the hands touch over head.
(4) Retain the breath a few minutes with hands over head.
(5) Lower hands slowly to sides, exhaling slowly at same time.
(6) Practice Cleansing Breath.

EXERCISE II.
(1) Stand erect, with arms straight In front of you.
(2) Inhale Complete Breath and retain.
(3) Swing arms back as far as they will go; then back to first position; then repeat several times, returning the breath all the while.
(4) Exhale vigorously through mouth.
(5) Practice Cleansing Breath.

EXERCISE III.
(1) Stand erect with arms straight In front of you,
(2) Inhale Complete Breath.
(3) Swing arms around in a circle, backward, a few times.
Then reverse a few times, retaining the breath all the while. You may vary this by rotating them alternately like the sails of a windmill.

(4) Exhale the breath vigorously through the mouth.
(5) Practice Cleansing Breath.

EXERCISE IV.
(1) Lie on the floor with your face downward and palms of hands flat upon the floor by your sides.
(2) Inhale Complete Breath and retain.
(3) Stiffen the body and raise yourself up by the strength of your arms until you rest on your hands and toes
(4) Then lower yourself to original position. Repeat several times.
(5) Exhale vigorously through your mouth.
(6) Practice Cleansing Breath.

EXERCISE V.
(1) Stand erect with your palms against the wall.

(2) Inhale Complete Breath and retain.
(3) Lower the chest to the wall, resting your weight on your hands.
(4) Then raise yourself back with the arm muscles alone, keeping the body stiff.
(5) Exhale vigorously through the mouth.
(6) Practice Cleansing Breath.

EXERCISE VI.

(1) Stand erect with arms "akimbo," that is, with hands resting around the waist and elbows standing out.
(2) Inhale Complete Breath and retain.
(3) Keep legs and hips stiff and bend well forward, as If bowing, at the same time exhaling slowly.
(4) Return to first position and take another Complete Breath.
(5) Then bend backward, exhaling slowly.
(6) Return to first position and take a Complete Breath.
(7) Then bend sideways, exhaling slowly. (Vary by bending to right and then to left.)
(8) Practice Cleansing Breath.

EXERCISE VII.

(1) Stand erect, or sit erect, with straight spinal column.
(2) Inhale a Complete Breath, but instead of inhaling in a continuous steady stream, take a series of short, quick "sniffs," as if you were smelling aromatic salts or ammonia and did not wish to get too strong a "whiff." Do not exhale any of these little breaths, but add one to the other until the entire lung space Is filled.
(3) Retain for a few seconds.
(4) Exhale through the nostrils in a long, restful, sighing breath.
(5) Practice Cleansing Breath.

CHAPTER XIII.

VIBRATION AND YOGI RHYTHMIC BREATHING

All is in vibration. From the tiniest atom to the greatest sun, everything is in a state of vibration. There is nothing in absolute rest in nature. A single atom deprived of vibration would wreck the universe. In incessant vibration the universal work is performed. Matter is being constantly played upon by energy and countless forms and numberless varieties result, and yet even the forms and varieties are not permanent. They begin to change the moment they are created, and from them are born innumerable forms, which in turn change and give rise to newer forms, and so on and on, in infinite succession. Nothing is permanent in the world of forms, and yet the great Reality is unchangeable. Forms are but appearances—they come, they go, but the Reality is eternal and unchangeable.

The atoms of the human body are in constant vibration. Unceasing changes are occurring. In a few months there is almost a complete change in the matter composing the body, and scarcely a single atom now composing your body will be found in It a few months hence. Vibration, constant vibration. Change, constant change.

In all vibration is to be found a certain rhythm. Rhythm pervades the universe. The swing of the planets around the sun; the rise and fall of the sea; the beating of the heart; the ebb and flow of the tide; all follow rhythmics laws. The rays of the sun reach us; the rain descends upon us, in obedience to the same law. All growth is but an exhibition of this law. All motion is a manifestation of the law of rhythm.

Our bodies are as much subject to rhythmic laws as is the planet in its revolution around the sun. Much of the esoteric side of the Yogi Science of Breath is based upon this known principle of nature. By falling in with the rhythm of the body, the Yogi manages to absorb a great amount of Prana, which he disposes of to bring about results desired by him. We will speak of this at greater length later on.

The body which you occupy is like a small inlet running in to the land from the sea. Although apparently subject only to its own laws, it is really subject to the ebb and flow of the tides of the ocean. The great sea of life is swelling and receding, rising and falling, and we are responding to its vibrations and rhythm. In a normal condition we receive the vibration and rhythm of the great ocean of life, and respond to it, but at times the mouth of the inlet seems choked up with debris, and we fail to receive the impulse from Mother Ocean, and inharmony manifests within us.

You have heard how a note on a violin, if sounded repeatedly and in rhythm, will start into motion vibrations which will in time destroy a bridge. The same result is true when a regiment of soldiers crosses a bridge, the order being always given to "break step" on such an occasion, lest the vibration bring down both bridge and regiment. These manifestations of the effect of rhythmic motion will give you an idea of the effect on the body of rhythmic breathing. The whole system catches the vibration and becomes in harmony with the will, which causes the rhythmic motion of the lungs, and while in such complete harmony will respond readily to orders from the will. With the body thus attuned, the Yogi finds no difficulty in increasing the circulation in any part of the body by an order from the will, and in the same way he can direct an increased current of nerve force to any part or organ, strengthening and stimulating it.

In the same way the Yogi by rhythmic breathing "catches the swing," as it were, and is able to absorb and control a greatly increased amount of prana, which is then at the disposal of his will. He can and does use it as a vehicle for sending forth thoughts to others and for attracting to him all those whose thoughts are keyed in the same vibration. The phenomena of telepathy, thought transference, mental healing, mesmerism, etc., which subjects are creating such an interest in the Western world at the present time, but which have been known to the Yogis for centuries, can be greatly increased and augmented If the person sending forth the thoughts will do so after rhythmic breathing. Rhythmic breathing will increase the value of mental healing, magnetic healing, etc., several hundred per cent.

In rhythmic breathing the main thing to be acquired is the mental idea of rhythm. To those who know anything of music, the idea of measured counting is familiar. To others, the rhythmic step of the soldier:

"Left, right; left, right; left, right; one, two, three, four; one, two, three, four," will convey the idea.

The Yogi bases his rhythmic time upon a unit corresponding with the beat of his heart. The heart beat varies in different persons, but the heart beat unit of each person is the proper rhythmic standard for that particular individual in his rhythmic breathing. Ascertain your normal heart beat by placing your fingers over your pulse, and then count: "1, 2, 3, 4, 5, 6; 1, 2, 3, 4, 5, 6," etc., until the rhythm becomes firmly fixed in your mind. A little practice will fix the rhythm, so that you will be able to easily reproduce it. The beginner usually inhales in about six pulse units, but he will be able to greatly increase this by practice.

The Yogi rule for rhythmic breathing is that the units of inhalation and exhalation should be the same, while the units for retention and between breaths should be one-half the number of those of inhalation and exhalation.

The following exercise in Rhythmic Breathing should be thoroughly

mastered, as it forms the basis of numerous other exercises, to which

reference will be made later.

---

(1) Sit erect, in an easy posture, being sure to hold the chest, neck and head as nearly in a straight line as possible, with shoulders slightly thrown back and hands resting easily on the lap. In this position the weight of the body is largely supported by the ribs and the position may be easily maintained. The Yogi has found that one cannot get the best effect of rhythmic breathing with the chest drawn in and the abdomen protruding.
(2) Inhale slowly a Complete Breath, counting six pulse units.
(3) Retain, counting three pulse units.
(4) Exhale slowly through the nostrils, counting six pulse units.
(5) Count three pulse beats between breaths.
(6) Repeat a number of times, but avoid fatiguing yourself at the start.
(7) When you are ready to close the exercise, practice the cleansing breath, which will rest you and cleanse the lungs.

After a little practice you will be able to increase the duration of the inhalations and exhalations, until about fifteen pulse units are consumed. In this increase, remember that the units for retention and between breaths is one-half the units for inhalation and exhalation.

Do not overdo yourself in your effort to increase the duration of the breath, but pay as much attention as possible to acquiring the "rhythm," as that is more important than the length of the breath. Practice and try until you get the measured "swing" of the movement, and until you can almost "feel" the rhythm of the vibratory motion throughout your whole body. It will require a little practice and perseverance, but your pleasure at your improvement will make the task an easy one. The Yogi is a most patient and persevering man, and his great attainments are due largely to the possession of these qualities.

CHAPTER XIV.

PHENOMENA OF YOGI PSYCHIC BREATHING.

With the exception of the instructions in the Yogi Rhythmic Breathing, the majority of the exercises heretofore given in this book relate to the physical plane of effort, which, while highly important in itself, is also regarded by the Yogis as in the nature of affording a substantial basis for efforts on the psychic and spiritual plane. Do not, however, discard or think lightly of the physical phase of the subject, for remember that it needs a sound body to support a sound mind, and also that the body is the temple of the Ego, the lamp in which burns the light of the Spirit. Everything is good in its place, and everything has its place. The developed man is the "all-around man," who recognizes body, mind and spirit and renders to each its due. Neglect of either is a mistake which must be rectified sooner or later; a debt which must be repaid with interest.

We will now take up the Psychic phase of the Yogi Science of Breath in the shape of a series of exercises, each exercise carrying with it its explanation.

You will notice that in each exercise rhythmic breathing is accompanied with the instructions to "carry the thought" of certain desired results. This mental attitude gives the Will a cleared track upon which to exercise its force. We cannot, in this work, go into the subject of the power of the Will, and must assume that you have some knowledge of the subject. If you have no acquaintance with the subject, you will find that the actual practice of the exercises themselves will give you a much clearer knowledge than any amount of theoretical teaching, for as the old Hindu proverb says, "He who tastes a grain of mustard seed knows more of its flavor than he who sees an elephant load of it."

(1)   GENERAL DIRECTIONS FOR YOGI PSYCHIC BREATHING.

The basis of all Yogi Psychic Breathing is the Yogi Rhythmic Breath, instruction regarding which we gave in our last chapter. In the following exercises, in order to avoid useless repetition, we will say merely, "Breathe Rhythmically," and then give the instruction for the exercise of the psychic force, or directed Will power working in connection with the rhythmic breath vibrations. After a little practice you will find that you will not need to count after the first rhythmic breath, as the mind will grasp the idea of time and rhythm and you will be able to breathe rhythmically at pleasure, almost automatically. This will leave the mind clear for the sending of the psychic vibrations under the direction of the Will. (See the following first exercise for directions in using the Will.)

(2)   PRANA DISTRIBUTING.

Lying flat on the floor or bed, completely relaxed, with hands resting lightly over the Solar Plexus (over the pit of the stomach, where the ribs begin to separate), breathe rhythmically. After the rhythm is fully established *will* that each inhalation will draw in an increased supply of prana or vital energy from the Universal supply, which will be taken up by the nervous system and stored in the Solar Plexus. At each exhalation will that the prana or vital energy is being distributed all over the body, to every organ and part; to every muscle, cell and atom; to nerve, artery and vein; from the top of your head to the soles of your feet; invigorating, strengthening and stimulating every nerve; recharging every nerve center; sending energy, force and strength all over the system. While exercising the will, try to form a mental picture of the inrushing prana, coming in through the lungs and being taken up at once by the Solar Plexus, then with the exhaling effort, being sent to all parts of the system, down to the finger tips and down to the toes. It is not necessary to use the Will with an effort. Simply commanding that which you wish to produce and then making the mental picture of it is all that is necessary. Calm command with the mental picture is far better than forcible willing, which only dissipates force needlessly. The above exercise is most helpful and greatly refreshes and strengthens the nervous system and produces a restful feeling all over the body. It is especially beneficial In cases where one is tired or feels a lack of energy.

(3) INHIBITING PAIN.

Lying down or sitting erect, breath rhythmically, holding the thought that you are inhaling prana. Then when you exhale, send the prana to the painful part to re-establish the circulation and nerve current. Then inhale more prana for the purpose of driving out the painful condition; then exhale, holding the thought that you are driving out the pain. Alternate the two above mental commands, and with one exhalation stimulate the part and with the next drive out the pain. Keep this up for seven breaths, then practice the Cleansing Breath and rest a while. Then try it again until relief comes, which will be before long. Many pains will be found to be relieved before the seven breaths are finished. If the hand is placed over the painful part, you may get quicker results. Send the current of prana down the arm and into the painful part.

(4) DIRECTING THE CIRCULATION.

Lying down or sitting erect, breathe rhythmically, and with the exhalations direct the circulation to any part you wish, which may be suffering from imperfect circulation. This is effective in cases of cold feet or in cases of headache, the blood being sent downward in both cases, in the first case warming the feet, and in the latter, relieving the brain from too great pressure. In the case of headache, try the Pain Inhibiting first, then follow with sending the blood downward. You will often feel a warm feeling in the legs as the circulation moves downward. The circulation is largely under the control of the will and rhythmic breathing renders the task easier.

(5)   SELF-HEALING.

Lying in a relaxed condition, breathe rhythmically, and command that a good supply of prana be inhaled. With the exhalation, send the prana to the affected part for the purpose of stimulating it. Vary this occasionally by exhaling, with the mental command that the diseased condition be forced out and disappear. Use the hands in this exercise, passing them down the body from the head to the affected part. In using the hands in healing yourself or others always hold the mental image that the prana is flowing down the arm and through the finger tips into the body, thus reaching the affected part and healing it. Of course we can give only general directions in this book without taking up the several forms of disease in detail, but a little practice of the above exercise, varying it slightly to fit the conditions of the case, will produce wonderful results. Some Yogis follow the plan of placing both hands on the affected part, and then breathing rhythmically, holding the mental image that they are fairly pumping prana into the diseased organ and part, stimulating it and driving out diseased conditions, as pumping into a pail of dirty water will drive out the latter and fill the bucket with fresh water. This last plan is very effective if the mental image of the pump is clearly held, the inhalation representing the lifting of the pump handle and the exhalation the actual pumping.

(6)   HEALING OTHERS.

We cannot take up the question of the psychic treatment of disease by prana in detail in this book, as such would be foreign to its purpose. But we can and will give you simple, plain instructions whereby you may be enabled to do much good in relieving others. The main principle to remember is that by rhythmic breathing and controlled thought you are enabled to absorb a considerable amount of prana, and are also able to pass it into the body of another person, stimulating weakened parts and organs and imparting health and driving out diseased conditions.

You must first learn to form such a clear mental image of the desired condition that you will be able to actually feel the influx of prana, and the force running down your arms and out of your finger tips into the body of the patient. Breathe rhythmically a few times until the rhythm is fairly established, then place your bands upon the affected part of the body of the patient, letting them rest lightly over the part. Then follow the "pumping" process described to the preceding exercise (Self-Healing) and fill the patient full of prana until the diseased condition is driven out. Every once in a while raise the hands and "flick" the fingers as if you were throwing off the diseased condition. It is well to do this occasionally and also to wash the hands after treatment, as otherwise you may take on a trace of the diseased condition of the patient.

Also practice the Cleansing Breath several times after the treatment. During the treatment let the prana pour into the patient in one continuous stream, allowing yourself to be merely the pumping machinery connecting the patient with the universal supply of prana, and allowing it to flow freely through you. You need not work the hands vigorously, but simply enough that the prana freely reaches the affected parts. The rhythmic breathing must be practiced frequently during the treatment, so as to keep the rhythm normal and to afford the prana a free passage. It is better to place the hands on the bare skin, but where this is not advisable or possible place them over the clothing.

Vary above method occasionally during the treatment by stroking the body gently and softly with the finger tips, the fingers being kept slightly separated. This is very soothing to the patient. In cases of long standing you may find it helpful to give the mental command in words, such as "get out, get out," or "be strong, be strong," as the case may be, the words helping you to exercise the will more forcibly and to the point. Vary these instructions to suit the needs of the case, and use your own judgment and inventive faculty. We have given you the general principles and you can apply them in hundreds of different ways. The above apparently simple instruction, if carefully studied and applied, will enable one to accomplish all that the leading "magnetic healers" are able to, although their "systems" are more or less cumbersome and complicated. They are using prana ignorantly and calling it "magnetism." If they would combine rhythmic breathing with their "magnetic" treatment they would double their efficiency.

(7)   DISTANT HEALING.

Prana colored by the thought of the sender may be projected to persons at a distance, who are willing to receive it, and healing work done in this way. This is the secret of the "absent healing," of which the Western world has heard so much of late years. The thought of the healer sends forth and colors the prana of the sender, and it flashes across space and finds lodgment in the psychic mechanism of the patient. It is unseen, and like the Marconi waves, it passes through intervening obstacles and seeks the person attuned to receive it. In order to treat persons at a distance, you must form a mental image of them until you can feel yourself to be en rapport with them. This is a psychic process dependent upon the mental imagery of the healer.

You can feel the sense of rapport when it is established, it manifesting in a sense of nearness. That is about as plain as we can describe it. It may be acquired by a little practice, and some will get it at the first trial. When rapport is established, say mentally to the distant patient, "I am sending you a supply of vital force or power, which will invigorate you and heal you." Then picture the prana as leaving your mind with each exhalation of rhythmic breath, and traveling across space instantaneously and reaching the patient and healing him. It is not necessary to fix certain hours for treatment, although you may do so if you wish. The receptive condition of the patient, as he is expecting and opening himself up to your psychic force, attunes him to receive your vibrations whenever you may send them. If you agree upon hours, let him place himself in a relaxed attitude and receptive condition. The above is the great underlying principle of the "absent treatment" of the Western world. You may do these things as well as the most noted healers, with a little practice.

CHAPTER XV.

MORE PHENOMENA OF YOGI PSYCHIC BREATHING.

(1)   THOUGHT PROJECTION.

Thoughts may be projected by following the last mentioned method (Distant Healing) and others will feel the effect of thought so sent forth, it being remembered always that no evil thought can ever injure another person whose thoughts are good. Good thoughts are always positive to bad ones, and bad ones always negative to good ones. One can, however, excite the interest and attention of another by sending him thought waves in this way, charging the prana with the message he wishes to convey. If you desire another's love and sympathy, and possess love and sympathy for him, you can send him thoughts of this kind with effect, providing your motives are pure. Never, however, attempt to influence another to his hurt, or from impure or selfish motives, as such thoughts only recoil upon the sender with redoubled force, and injure him, while the innocent party is not affected. Psychic force when legitimately used is all right, but beware of "black magic" or improper and unholy uses of it, as such attempts are like playing with a dynamo, and the person attempting such things will be surely punished by the result of the act itself. However, no person of impure motives ever acquires a great degree of psychic power, and a pure heart and mind is an invulnerable shield against improper psychic power. Keep yourself pure and nothing can hurt you.

(2)   FORMING AN AURA.

If you are ever in the company of persons of a low order of mind, and you feel the depressing influence of their thought, breathe rhythmically a few times, thus generating an additional supply of prana, and then by means of the mental image method surround yourself with an egg-shaped thought aura, which will protect you from the gross thought and disturbing influences of others.

(3)   RECHARGING YOURSELF.

If you feel that your vital energy is at a low ebb, and that you need to store up a new supply quickly, the best plan is to place the feet close together (side by side, of course) and to lock the fingers of both hands in any way that seems the most comfortable. This closes the circuit, as it were, and prevents any escape of prana through the extremities. Then breathe rhythmically a few times, and you will feel the effect of the recharging.

(4)   RECHARGING OTHERS.

If some friend is deficient in vitality you may aid him by sitting in front of him, your toes touching his, and his hands in yours. Then both breathe rhythmically, you forming the mental image of sending prana into his system, and he holding the mental image of receiving the prana. Persons of weak vitality or passive will should be careful with whom they try this experiment, as the prana of a person of evil desires will be colored with the thoughts of that person, and may give him a temporary influence over the weaker person. The latter, however, may easily remove such influence by closing the circuit (as before mentioned) and breathing a few rhythmic breaths, closing with the Cleansing Breath.

(5)   CHARGING WATER.

Water may be charged with prana, by breathing rhythmically, and holding the glass of water by the bottom, in the left hand, and then gathering the fingers of the right hand together and shaking them gently over the water, as if you were shaking drops of water off of your finger tips into the glass. The mental image of the prana being passed into the water must also be held. Water thus charged is found stimulating to weak or sick persons, particularly if a healing thought accompanies the mental image of the transfer of the prana. The caution given in the last exercise applies also to this one, although the danger exists only in a greatly lessened degree.

(6)   ACQUIRING MENTAL QUALITIES.

Not only can the body be controlled by the mind under direction of the will, but the mind itself can be trained and cultivated by the exercise of the controlling will. This, which the Western world knows as "Mental Science," etc., has proved to the West portions of that truth which the Yogi has known for ages. The mere calm demand of the Will will accomplish wonders in this direction, but if the mental exercise is accompanied by rhythmic breathing, the effect is greatly increased. Desirable qualities may be acquired by holding the proper mental image of what is desired during rhythmic breathing. Poise and Self Control, desirable qualities; increased power, etc., may be acquired in this way. Undesirable qualities may be eliminated by cultivating the opposite qualities. Any or all the "Mental Science" exercises, "treatments" and "affirmations" may be used with the Yogi Rhythmic Breath. The following is a good general exercise for the acquirement and development of desirable mental qualities:

Lie in a passive attitude, or sit erect. Picture to yourself the qualities you desire to cultivate, seeing yourself as possessed of the qualities, and demanding that your mind develop the quality. Breathe rhythmically, holding the mental picture firmly. Carry the mental picture with you as much as possible, and endeavor to live up to the ideal you have set up in your mind.

You will find yourself gradually growing up to your ideal. The rhythm of the breathing assists the mind in forming new combinations, and the student who has followed the Western system will find the Yogi Rhythmic a wonderful ally in his "Mental Science" works.

(7)   ACQUIRING PHYSICAL QUALITIES.

Physical qualities may be acquired by the same methods as above mentioned in connection with mental qualities. We do not mean, of course, that short men can be made tall, or that amputated limbs may be replaced, or similar miracles. But the expression of the countenance may be changed; courage and general physical characteristics improved by the control of the Will, accompanied by rhythmic breathing. As a man thinks so does he look, act, walk, sit, etc. Improved thinking will mean improved looks and actions. To develop any part of the body, direct the attention to it, while breathing rhythmically, holding the mental picture that you are sending an increased amount of prana, or nerve force, to the part, and thus increasing its vitality and developing it. This plan applies equally well to any part of the body which you wish to develop. Many Western athletes use a modification of this plan in their exercises. The student who has followed our instructions so far will readily understand haw to apply the Yogi principles in the above work. The general rule of exercise is the same as in the preceding exercise (acquiring Mental Qualities). We have touched upon the subject of the cure of physical ailments in preceding pages.

(8)   CONTROLLING THE EMOTIONS.

The undesirable emotions, such as Fear, Worry, Anxiety, Hate, Anger, Jealousy, Envy, Melancholy, Excitement, Grief, etc., are amenable to the control of the Will, and the Will is enabled to operate more easily in such cases if rhythmic breathing is practiced while the student is "willing." The following exercise has been found most effective by the Yogi students, although the advanced Yogi has but little need of it, as he has long since gotten rid of these undesirable mental qualities by growing spiritually beyond them. The Yogi student, however, finds the exercise a great help to him while he is growing.

Breathe rhythmically, concentrating the attention upon the Solar Plexus, and sending to it the mental command "Get Out." Send the mental command firmly, just as you begin to exhale, and form the mental picture of the undesirable emotions being carried away with the exhaled breath. Repeat seven times, and finish with the Cleansing Breath, and then see how good you feel. The mental command must be given "in earnest," as trifling will not do the work.

(9)   TRANSMUTATION OF THE REPRODUCTIVE ENERGY.

The Last Weight-loss Program You Will Ever Need

The Yogis possess great knowledge regarding the use and abuse of the reproductive principle in both sexes. Some hints of this esoteric knowledge have filtered out and have been used by Western writers on the subject, and much good has been accomplished in this way. In this little book we cannot do more than touch upon the subject, and omitting all except a bare mention of theory, we will give a practical breathing exercise whereby the student will be enabled to transmute the reproductive energy into vitality for the entire system, instead of dissipating and wasting it in lustful indulgences in or out of the marriage relations. The reproductive energy is creative energy, and may be taken up by the system and transmuted into strength and vitality, thus serving the purpose of regeneration instead of generation. If the young men of the Western world understood these underlying principles they would be saved much misery and unhappiness in after years, and would be stronger mentally, morally and physically.

This transmutation of the reproductive energy gives great vitality to those practicing it. They will be filled with great vital force, which will radiate from them and will manifest in what has been called "personal magnetism." The energy thus transmuted may be turned into new channels and used to great advantage. Nature has condensed one of its most powerful manifestations of prana into reproductive energy, as its purpose is to create. The greatest amount of vital force is concentrated in the smallest area. The reproductive organism is the most powerful storage battery in animal life, and its force can be drawn upward and used, as well as expended in the ordinary functions of reproduction, or wasted in riotous lust. The majority of our students know something of the theories of regeneration; and we can do little more than to state the above facts, without attempting to prove them.

The Yogi exercise for transmuting reproductive energy is simple. It is coupled with rhythmic breathing, and can be easily performed. It may be practiced at any time, but is specially recommended when one feels the instinct most strongly, at which time the reproductive energy is manifesting and may be most easily transmuted for regenerative purposes. The exercise is as follows: Keep the mind fixed on the idea of Energy, and away from ordinary sexual thoughts or imaginings. If these thoughts come into the mind do not be discouraged, but regard them as manifestations of a force which you intend using for the purposes of strengthening the body and mind. Lie passively or sit erect, and fix your mind on the idea of drawing the reproductive energy upward to the Solar Plexus, where it will be transmuted and stored away as a reserve force of vital energy. Then breathe rhythmically, forming the mental image of drawing up the reproductive energy with each inhalation. With each inhalation make a command of the Will that the energy be drawn upward from the reproductive organization to the Solar Plexus. If the rhythm is fairly established and the mental image is clear, you will be conscious of the upward passage of the energy, and will feel its stimulating effect. If you desire an increase in mental force, you may draw it up to the brain instead of to the Solar Plexus, by giving the mental command and holding the mental image of the transmission to the brain. The man or woman doing metal creative work, or bodily creative work, will be able to use this creative energy in their work by following the above exercise, drawing up the energy with the inhalation and sending it forth with the exhalation. In this last form of exercise, only such portions as are needed in the work will pass into the work being done, the balance remaining stored up in the Solar Plexus. You will understand, of course, that it is not the reproductive fluids which are drawn up and used, but the etheripranic energy which animates the latter, the soul of the reproductive organism, as it were. It is usual to allow the head to bend forward easily and naturally during the transmuting exercise.

(10)   BRAIN STIMULATING.

The Yogis have found the following exercise most useful in stimulating the action of the brain for the purpose of producing clear thinking and reasoning. It has a wonderful effect in clearing the brain and nervous system, and those engaged in mental work will find it most useful to them, both in the direction of enabling them to do better work and also as a means of refreshing the mind and clearing it after arduous mental labor.

Sit in an erect posture, keeping the spinal column straight, and the eyes well to the front, letting the hands rest on the upper part of the legs. Breathe rhythmically, but instead of breathing through both nostrils as in the ordinary exercises, press the left nostril close with the thumb, and inhale through the right nostril. Then remove the thumb, and close the right nostril with the finger, and then exhale through the left nostril. Then, without changing the fingers, inhale through the left nostril, and changing fingers, exhale through the right. Then inhale through right and exhale through left, and so on, alternating nostrils as above mentioned, closing the unused nostril with the thumb or forefinger. This is one of the oldest forms of Yogi breathing, and is quite important and valuable, and is well worthy of acquirement. But it is quite amusing to the Yogis to know that to the Western world this method is often held out as being the "whole secret" of Yogi Breathing. To the minds of many Western readers, "Yogi Breathing" suggests nothing more than a picture of a Hindu, sitting erect, and alternating nostrils in the act of breathing. "Only this and nothing more." We trust that this little work will open the eyes of the Western world to the great possibilities of Yogi Breathing, and the numerous methods whereby it may be employed.

(11)   THE GRAND YOGI PSYCHIC BREATH.

The Yogis have a favorite form of psychic breathing which they practice occasionally, to which has been given a Sanscrit term of which the above is a general equivalent. We have given it last, as it requires practice on the part of the student in the line of rhythmic breathing and mental imagery, which he has now acquired by means of the preceding exercises. The general principles of the Grand Breath may be summed up in the old Hindu saying: "Blessed is the Yogi who can breathe through his bones." This exercise will fill the entire system with prana, and the student will emerge from it with every bone, muscle, nerve, cell, tissue, organ and part energized and attuned by the prana and the rhythm of the breath. It is a general housecleaning of the system, and he who practices it carefully will feel as if he had been given a new body, freshly created, from the crown of his head to the tips of his toes. We will let the exercise speak for itself.

(1) Lie in a relaxed position, at perfect ease.
(2) Breathe rhythmically until the rhythm is perfectly established.
(3) Then, inhaling and exhaling, form the mental image of the breath being drawn up through the bones of the legs, and then forced out through them; then through the bones of the arms; then through the top of the skull; then through the stomach; then through the reproductive region; then as if it were traveling upward and downward along the spinal column; and then as if the breath were being inhaled and exhaled through every pore of the skin, the whole body being filled with prana and life.
(4) Then (breathing rhythmically) send the current of prana to the Seven Vital Centers, in turn, as follows, using the mental picture as in previous exercises:

   (a) To the forehead.
   (b) To the back of the head.
   (c) To the base of the brain.
   (d) To the Solar Plexus.
   (e) To the Sacral Region (lower part of the spine).
   (f) To the region of the navel.
   (g) To the reproductive region.

Finish by sweeping the current of prana, to and fro from head to feet several times.
(5) Finish with Cleansing Breath.

CHAPTER XVI.

YOGI SPIRITUAL BREATHING.

The Yogis not only bring about desired mental qualities and properties by will-power coupled with rhythmic breathing, but they also develop spiritual faculties, or rather aid in their unfoldment, in the same way. The Oriental philosophies teach that man has many faculties which are at present in a dormant state, but which will become unfolded as the race progresses. They also teach that man, by the proper effort of the will, aided by favorable conditions, may aid in the unfoldment of these spiritual faculties, and develop them much sooner than in the ordinary process of evolution. In other words, one may even now develop spiritual powers of consciousness which will not become the common property of the race until after long ages of gradual development under the law of evolution. In all of the exercises directed toward this end, rhythmic breathing plays an important part. There is of course no mystic property in the breath itself which produces such wonderful results, but the rhythm produced by the Yogi breath is such as to bring the whole system, including the brain, under perfect control, and in perfect harmony, and by this means, the most perfect condition is obtained for the unfoldment of these latent faculties.

In this work we cannot go deeply into the philosophy of the East regarding spiritual development, because this subject would require volumes to cover it, and then again the subject is too abstruse to interest the average reader. There are also other reasons, well known to occultists, why this knowledge should not be spread broadcast at this time. Rest assured, dear student, that when the time comes for you to take the next step, the way will be opened out before you. "When the chela (student) is ready, the guru (master) appears." In this chapter we will give you directions for the development of two phases of spiritual consciousness, i.e., (1) the consciousness of the identity of the Soul, and (2) the consciousness of the connection of the Soul with the Universal Life. Both of the exercises given below are simple, and consist of mental images firmly held, accompanied with rhythmic breathing. The student must not expect too much at the start, but must make haste slowly, and be content to develop as does the flower, from seed to blossom.

SOUL CONSCIOUSNESS.
The real Self is not the body or even the mind of man. These things are but a part of his personality, the lesser self. The real Self is the Ego, whose manifestation is in individuality. The real Self is independent of the body, which it inhabits, and is even independent of the mechanism of the mind, which it uses as an instrument. The real Self is a drop from the Divine Ocean, and is eternal and indestructible. It cannot die or be annihilated, and no matter what becomes of the body, the real Self still exists. It is the Soul. Do not think of your Soul as a thing apart from you, for YOU are the Soul, and the body is the unreal and transitory part of you which is changing in material every day, and which you will some day discard. You may develop the faculties so that they will be conscious of the reality of the Soul, and its independence of the body. The Yogi plan for such

development is by meditation upon the real Self or Soul, accompanied by rhythmic breathing. The following exercise is the simplest form.

EXERCISE.—Place your body in a relaxed, reclining position. Breathe rhythmically, and meditate upon the real Self, thinking of yourself as an entity independent of the body, although inhabiting it and being able to leave it at will. Think of yourself, not as the body, but as a spirit, and of your body as but a shell, useful and comfortable, but not a part of the real You. Think of yourself as an independent being, using the body only as a convenience. While meditating, ignore the body entirely, and you will find that you will often become almost entirely unconscious of it, and will seem to be out of the body to which you may return when you are through with the exercise.

This is the gist of the Yogi meditative breathing methods, and if persisted in will give one a wonderful sense of the reality of the Soul, and will make him seem almost independent of the body. The sense of immortality will often come with this increased consciousness, and the person will begin to show signs of spiritual development which will be noticeable to himself and others. But he must not allow himself to live too much in the upper regions, or to despise his body, for he is here on this plane for a purpose, and he must not neglect his opportunity to gain the experiences necessary to round him out, nor must he fail to respect his body, which is the Temple of the Spirit.

THE UNIVERSAL CONSCIOUSNESS.
The Spirit in man, which is the highest manifestation of his Soul, is a drop in the ocean of Spirit, apparently separate and distinct, but yet really in touch with the ocean itself, and with every other drop in it. As man unfolds in spiritual consciousness he becomes more and more aware of his relation to the Universal Spirit, or Universal Mind as some term it. He feels at times as if he were almost at-one-ment with it, and then again he loses the sense of contact and relationship.

The Yogis seek to attain this state of Universal Consciousness by meditation and rhythmic breathing, and many have thus attained the highest degree of spiritual attainment possible to man in this stage of his existence. The student of this work will not need the higher instruction regarding adeptship at this time, as he has much to do and accomplish before he reaches that stage, but it may be well to initiate him into the elementary stages of the Yogi exercises for developing Universal Consciousness, and if he is in earnest he will discover means and methods whereby he may progress. The way is always opened to him who is ready to tread the path. The following exercise will be found to do much toward developing the Universal Consciousness in those who faithfully practice it.

EXERCISE.—Place your body in a reclining, relaxed position. Breathe rhythmically, and meditate upon your relationship with the Universal Mind of which you are but an atom. Think of yourself as being in touch with All, and at-one-ment with All. See All as One, and your Soul as a part of that One. Feel that you are receiving the vibrations from the great Universal Mind, and are partaking of its power and strength and wisdom. The two following lines of meditation may be followed.

(a) With each inhalation, think of yourself as drawing in to yourself the strength and power of the Universal Mind. When exhaling think of yourself as passing out to others that same power, at the same time being filled with love for every living thing, and desiring that it be a partaker of the same blessings which you are now receiving. Let the Universal Power circulate through you.

(b) Place your mind in a reverential state, and meditate upon the grandeur of the Universal Mind, and open yourself to the inflow of the Divine Wisdom, which will fill you with illuminating wisdom, and then let the same flow out from you to your brothers and sisters whom you love and would help.

This exercise leaves with those who have practiced it a new-found sense of strength, power and wisdom, and a feeling of spiritual exaltation and bliss. It must be practiced only in a serious, reverential mood, and must not be approached triflingly or lightly.

GENERAL DIRECTIONS.

The exercises given in this chapter require the proper mental attitude and conditions, and the trifler and person of a non-serious nature, or one without a sense of spirituality and reverence, had better pass them by, as no results will be obtained by such persons, and besides it is a wilful trifling with things of a high order, which course never benefits those who pursue it. These exercises are for the few who can understand them, and the others will feel no attraction to try them.

During meditation let the mind dwell upon the ideas given in the exercise, until it becomes clear to the mind, and gradually manifests in real consciousness within you. The mind will gradually become passive and at rest, and the mental image will manifest clearly. Do not indulge in these exercises too often, and do not allow the blissful state produced to render you dissatisfied with the affairs of everyday life, as the latter are useful and necessary for you, and you must never shirk a lesson, however disagreeable to you it may be. Let the joy arising from the unfolding consciousness buoy you up and nerve you for the trials of life, and not make you dissatisfied and disgusted. All is good, and everything has its place.

The Last Weight-loss Program You Will Ever Need

Many of the students who practice these exercises will in time wish to know more. Rest assured that when the time comes we will see that you do not seek in vain. Go on in courage and confidence, keeping your face toward the East, from whence comes the rising Sun.

Peace be unto you, and unto all men.

■ ■

END OF BOOK.

We really hope you have benefited from this book. Please email us at Dr.More a t- drmoreu2@gmail.com and we are standing by to help you, in any small way we can. God Bless!

We run a weight-loss membership program. Please check it out. Website is below.

Dr.Morgan.

www.weightloss-expert-group.com

www.ingramcontent.com/pod-product-compliance
Lightning Source LLC
Chambersburg PA
CBHW070651290526
45790CB00001B/272